Life With Mike

ANGIE R. DOUTHIT

⊕ **Strategic Book Publishing**

Strategic Book Publishing
An imprint of Strategic Book Group
P.O.Box 333
Durham, CT 06422

www.StrategicBookGroup.com

ISBN: 978-1-60911-120-5

Printed in the United States of America

To Michael Patrick Williams "Douthit": My hero, my biggest fan, my encourager, my buddy, and my son. Our lives changed forever the day we began caring for you. Because of you, we are now rich beyond words, not with money, but with a deep revelation of how God can take a life that the world might see as a mistake, and turn it into perfection. Mike, you were the most loving, kind, generous, understanding person I have ever known. We all miss you. We will forever remember you.

Also, to my husband Brad, and our children, Whitney, Kaylee, Zeke, and Mackenzie; you never questioned why we were taking care of Mike. You all knew it was God's purpose for us to share our lives with him. I know how much you loved him and how we are better human beings because of our life with Mike.

And to God, my father and Savior, thank you for allowing us to share seventeen years with Mike and for allowing us to be at his bedside when you carried him into Glory.

Contents

Preface

I wish you all could have met Mike. Actually, a person did not meet Mike, they experienced him. You see, Mike lived with Down's syndrome, yet in his own unique way, he demonstrated how we should live our lives. He loved God. He loved family. He believed life was precious. He adored elderly people. He loved children, animals, and hugs. He loved food. He loved Republicans. And, he loved living life together with friends and family. Just talking with Mike made you feel better. He made you laugh, and he made you stop and see that life was not all about getting ahead and being successful. He taught us that life was about being happy, loving Jesus, and eating good food.

In reading his story, you will see that Mike was not handicapped in the traditions of the world. He was a truly amazing person with wonderful lessons to teach those who knew him. As you read Mike's story, I trust you will be led to a more personal glimpse of the Savior that Mike adored. I also pray you will view *all* life as precious and as having a purpose. God does not make mistakes and he sure knew what he was doing when he brought Mike into our lives. I think of Mike daily. Sometimes I cry, sometimes I laugh, and sometimes I just look around the house and thank God for our *Life With Mike.*

Angie Douthit
Miami, Oklahoma

Special Thanks

I asked God to provide an editor for this book that knew and understood Mike. God used my uncle, Dr. Robert Lee Wilson, Director of Missions for Enon Baptist Association of Oklahoma. Thank you, Uncle Robert. Deanne Garrison, the director of women's ministries for EBA and retired English composition teacher, also aided in the editing and revising of this book. I highly appreciate the time you spent editing. May God bless you both mightily!

Chapter 1

The Miracle of Being Together

Mike's family moved him into a group home following his mother's sudden death; his father had disappeared shortly after his birth and his family was not able to care for him. My husband Brad and I went to visit Mike at the group home before he came to live with us. I will always remember seeing Mike for the first time. He was adorable. He was short, about 5 feet 5 inches and weighed around 145 pounds. His hair was thin, straight, and brown, and he parted it to the side and brushed it over. He pulled his shorts up to his rib cage, tucked his shirts in, and always wore a belt. He pulled his striped socks up to his knees. His arms were shorter than most peoples' and his belly protruded. His smile was infectious, with his crooked teeth and thin lips. He would tilt his head to the side and smile and bat his eyelashes at you. He reminded me of a loving puppy with whom you instantly fell in love. He extended his short, plump arms for a hug. I was hooked.

It was rather scary at the group home and I will never forget Mike looking at me with his wild right eye, and whispering in my ear, "These people here are crazy!" After a few minutes there, I totally agreed with him. You could not determine who was an employee and who was a patient as they all came and talked to you and asked you your name. Mike did not belong there. He had been raised in society and was used to the normal flow of life. After spending some time with him, Brad and I knew we were the family to take care of him.

A few weeks later, Mike came and spent his first weekend with us. He entertained us by telling fictional stories about siblings that he never had. He had Brad and me crying, as he told us, in detail, about his little sister with blond curly hair, who died when she choked on a chicken bone, and about his little brother wearing overalls, who had died of pneumonia. We felt so sorry for him and our hearts ached for this sweet little man telling us these tragic stories. We later found out that he was an only child and fabricated the stories. We also discovered later that he had badly wanted brothers and sisters and had often prayed for them. His detailed stories were probably reflections of his dreams.

A huge TV buff, he loved the *Partridge Family* so much that he had actually contacted Danny Bonaduce, a star of the show, by phone. Danny had missed Mike's call, so he called him back. His birth mother had answered the phone. When she realized Danny Bonaduce was on the other line, it scared her and she hung up. His mother, totally shocked by the phone call, realized how much Mike wanted a big family.

As I later pondered over our first weekend with Mike and how he had told us the made-up stories, I realized how intensely he had always wanted siblings. God had granted his wish by making Mike part of our family. Mike was finally going to have sisters and later, a brother. He was very delighted and proud, and we were truly blessed.

Chapter 2

Foster Parenting

Brad and I have had an interesting life. We truly were "high school sweethearts." We fell in love at his freshmen end-of-year school dance. He was fifteen and I was fourteen. We knew right away that we wanted to marry one day and spend the rest of our lives together. We both wanted a big family, as we both loved children. We married in 1987. Our first child, Whitney, was born in October of that year. Our second child, Kaylee, was born three and a half years later in March of 1991. We were happy and busy.

Our young family lived in a mobile home in the country. Whitney loved the country and we felt that we would live there for our entire married life. It was a great location, but the trailer needed some major repair. When it rained you needed an umbrella if you stood by the windows. This mobile home was an older one that had a metal roof. The windows leaked badly, which caused all of the windowsills to rot away. Brad was working at a factory and I stayed home with the girls and babysat for my friend.

Brad and I began to feel God calling us to become foster parents. We loved children and wanted to share our lives with those who needed love. We knew that our trailer would not pass state inspection for foster parenting, so we began praying for a house. I filled out the papers to have a small house built on our land, which was owned by Brad's dad. When the home loan was approved, his dad decided not to let us build on his land. We were confused and frustrated and sought the Lord's will. I will never forget the day my dad called and asked if we were interested in taking care of a man with Down's syndrome. "Oh yeah," he said. "His mother has a home that she built for him. She passed away, and his family wants someone to live in the home and take care of him." When Brad and I had decided to be foster parents, we had thought it would be for small children. We had never considered a grown man with mental retardation. The entire situation, however, sounded like a great big God thing. So we agreed to look at the house and to have Mike spend the weekend with us to see how we all clicked.

The moment I stepped into the house I knew we were meant to be there. You see, I had prayed for a house for four years, and I had told God specific things that I wanted in a home. I wanted a separate living room and den. I wanted a sun porch for plants, and I wanted a big yard for my children to play in. Mike's house had every single one of those things with a few added items that I had not considered. I knew that God had built this house for my family to share with Mike. Brad and I were so thankful. Not only had God provided us with a wonderful home, he also gave us a son who would change our lives forever.

Chapter 3

Halloween Night

We moved into the house on October 26, 1991. Mike came to live with us on October 31, Halloween night. We took him trick-or-treating and introduced him to our families. Brad's mom was having a Halloween party. Mike walked in and right away began dancing, which was his hilarious version of "The Twist," laughing his loud infectious laugh, and greeting the family with hugs and a warm handshake. He acted as if he had known every one of them all of his life. He directly called our parents Grandma and Grandpa and our siblings were "aunt" and "uncle." Mike loved being at the party and beyond doubt enjoyed the food. It was a delightful night for all. We have talked and reflected often about our first extraordinary night with Mike.

The first months with Mike were quite an adjustment for me. Brad worked in a town sixty miles away and was gone Monday through Friday from 5:00 A.M. until 5:00 P.M. He was so exhausted when he got home that he collapsed in the recliner until bedtime. I was not used to having another adult in the house. Mike followed me around and talked nonstop. I was used to being with our two small children and found it strange to be entertaining another adult all the time. Mike and I soon became used to each other, and I grew to cherish our interesting conversations. He would tell me made-up stories and I would say, "Mike, you know that did not happen." He would respond with, "We'll see time comes." He always made me laugh and as time went by, I realized that Mike was an enormous help with my girls. He would sit at the kitchen table and bounce Kaylee and Whitney on his knee while I cooked and cleaned the dishes. He would also let them ride on his foot while he would sing, "Giddee up, horsee." They loved him, as he was very patient, kind, and gentle. It was so cute to see him sit on the floor with them and play Barbie's and work puzzles. Whitney would get out her Little Mermaid coloring books and Mike would color with her while she reminded him to stay in the lines. He could also stand and push the swing on the swing set for hours, which was how we got Kaylee to sleep most afternoons.

Mike functioned on a high level and could bathe, dress, and feed himself. He also had wonderful grooming skills. His mother must have worked on those skills because he had a great system. He would lay his pajamas on his bed, then get his robe, towel, and wash cloth. He would take them to the bathroom and start his bathwater. We would listen outside the door to him blowing bubbles in the water and splashing like a big fish in the tub. I loved to listen to him talk to himself. He would carry on an entire conversation and then laugh a hardy laugh. He would finish his laughter by saying, "You better watch that." He would then let out the water, dry off, and get dressed. He would walk out wearing pajamas, robe, and slippers. He would pull his pajama pants up to his rib cage and tuck in his shirt. He would also comb his hair over to the side and splash on some aftershave. Mike groomed himself better than most men I know. He would make his bed every day and knew how to put his clothes away in the drawers. He also knew how to match his clothes and loved to wear suits with a matching tie to church on Sundays.

We enjoyed seventeen more Halloween nights with Mike. He loved dressing up and treasured receiving candy. He smiled as he said, "Trick-or-Treat, give me something good to eat." He helped me pass out candy and enjoyed seeing the kids dressed in their costumes. He found it funny to yell, "BOO!" to everyone who rang our doorbell. He certainly knew how to make holidays entertaining.

Chapter 4

Church

Mike loved to go to church. He had been raised going to the First Assembly of God church. It was ironic, because the church I have attended since I was eight years old is a Southern Baptist church that purchased the building from the First Assembly of God church when they built a new building. Mike had accepted Christ as his savior and had been baptized in the same building where we now attended services. He loved both churches and often referred to himself as a "bapticostal." We let him attend the Assembly of God church for the first few years while we went to our Baptist church. Then he started asking to go with us. Our church family loved him and treated him wonderfully. They knew he loved Jesus and also our church dinners.

When we first started taking Mike to church, he did sign language to the music. He would raise his short, chubby arms in the air and make what looked like beautiful sign language. I was so proud of him as people would watch in amazement at how talented he was. However, in time we realized that Mike used the same four or five signs for everything we sang. No one minded. We knew he was praising the Lord in a language that only God and Mike understood.

Mike loved church on Wednesday nights because he got to go to

RAs. RA stands for Royal Ambassadors. It was a class for boys in first through sixth grade. My husband Brad helped teach the class with our good friend Chris. RAs is a class that studies sports and being active along with a lesson about Christ. Oh yes, and did I mention that they also had a snack? Mike loved going with Brad to class, he loved being with the little boys, and he loved the snacks. While the boys, Brad, and Chris were playing a sport game like basketball, football, or golf, Mike would stand on the sidelines cheering. He would raise his dumpy arms in the air and turn around in circles shouting, "Yeah daddy, yeah Uncle Chris, yeah Zeke, thank you good Lord, praise you Jesus." The little boys would laugh and give Mike a hug. They all loved him and he loved them back.

Then the snacks would be delivered. The boys were asked to form a line and wait their turn for a snack. Mike would try to be first in line but he wasn't quite fast enough. Brad and Chris realized how much he liked the snacks and would sometimes give Mike his snack last just to tease him. He would wait patiently and many times they would tell him that the snacks were all gone. He would make a sad face and say, "Don't say that, I hungry, I need food." With that they would laugh and give him his snack. Many times they would try to tease him by taking his snack away after he got it. He would fight back by using his version of karate. He would kick his leg in the air (about six inches off the ground) and give a karate chop into the air with his arm and say, "Haa-Yaa." It was quite humorous. If the karate did not work, he would lay his head on Chris' shoulder and say, "I love you, Uncle Chris." Mike's contagious smile and love won Chris over every time and Mike was given his snack.

Mike loved to sit by my grandma and grandpa during Sunday church services. He would look at me and say, "I sit by the nice old people, okay?" as he tilted his head to the side, batted his eyelashes at me, and grinned. It was hard to say no to a face like Mike's.

Mike quickly learned that if he coughed in church grandma

would give him a peppermint candy. Right after the singing was finished, you could hear Mike beginning his fake cough. Quiet at first, then a little louder, then before he could belt out a real loud one, Grandma would reach in her purse and hand him a peppermint. It was rather miraculous how quickly a peppermint could cure his cough. At least his breath smelled good when we were shaking hands and greeting new visitors.

Mike was often the source of humor in church. He loved the preaching and stated aloud many amusing comments during the sermons. If the preacher ever mentioned marriage, Mike would say very loudly "I get married." The crowd would snicker with quiet laughs. Mike said that he was getting married so many times that people learned to just shake their heads and agree with him by saying, "That's nice, Mike." He also loved to stand up during Mother's Day when they would recognize mothers. He would stand and say, "I getting married and I'm pregnant." Grandma would try to stop him but he was amazingly fast when he wanted to be. I will never forget the time Mike came dancing down the aisle during a congregational song and went straight down to the front near the podium. He was doing the "Mike boogie" right in front of God and everybody. I tried to reach him to stop him but it was too late. The teenagers, who sit in the front pew, were already out of control with laughter. I caught a glimpse of my daughter Kaylee as her face turned red from laughing so hard. I then looked at my daughter Whitney as tears rolled down her face from laughing so long. I shook my head at them because they were continuously encouraging Mike to dance for their friends. Now he was showing the church family his unique talent. The song leader just grinned and kept right on singing.

I do believe, however, that Mike's favorite thing about coming to church was the church dinners. Mike loved potluck dinners and always found a seat in the fellowship hall and awaited the wonderful plate I was filling just for him. People soon learned to let me get

Mike's plate first or he would begin asking compassionate women to get him something to eat. I would show up with his plate and he would already have a piece of cake and coffee. He would grin and say, "That lady so nice, she brought me dessert."

Mike would eat everything except carrots and red tomatoes; he would only eat yellow tomatoes, not red ones. I asked him why he did not eat red tomatoes and he told me that the acid would break his face out. I assumed he had been told that when he was a teenager and believed tomatoes would still break his face out. I never convinced him otherwise. Even Grandma tried to talk him into eating tomatoes and carrots, but he was very headstrong about the idea.

Mike knew to save his dessert for last. I suppose his mother had trained him to wait. A few men in the church realized how much he enjoyed food and began teasing him and giving him a hard time, pretending to take his plate of food or his dessert plate. During his younger years, Mike would laugh along with them. As he became older, however, he no longer found it funny and would try to stab them with his plastic fork if they came near his plate of dessert. He got so frustrated with one man in particular who kept teasing Mike, saying he was going to take his chocolate cake, that Mike looked at me and said "Mama, he's Satan!" We all roared with laughter and not long after, this nice man became known as "Satan" to several people in church. A few years later, when Mike was ill and in ICU, this man and his wife came to visit him. I said, "Hey Mike, Satan is here to see you." We all laughed remembering how much fun we'd had at the church dinners teasing Mike.

People at church adored Mike. As he got older and became slower in his walking, many of the teenagers would help him to the car. They would take his hand, walk him to our van, and help him into his favorite seat. He always sat in the same seat, right behind the passenger's seat. It is hard to look at that seat in our van now and not picture Mike sitting there, waving and blowing kisses to the "nice people" (as Mike referred to them) at church.

I always knew that Mike had a special link with God. He loved to pray, especially before meals. Mike would not take a bite of food until we prayed. Even if someone else started eating before the prayer, Mike would not take one bite. If you forgot to pray and everyone started eating, Mike would lower his head, close his eyes, and say his own prayer. It would make all sitting near him realize their selfishness and prompt them to bow their heads and pray also. His real mother had obviously raised him right. He would pray and thank God for everyone in the room and their pets. He never prayed for himself, though. I think he figured we needed it more. He would go on and on forever. I finally learned to say "Amen," and he would immediately say "Jesus name to thee, Amen."

There were many times over the years that we would be in the middle of a family crisis or a moment of being upset and fretful, and then I would realize Mike was missing. I would always find him on his knees, next to his bed. With his hands folded in prayer, and his eyes raised toward heaven, Mike would be praying out loud, "Lord Jesus please help my mama and Lord Jesus help my daddy and please help my sisters and my brother in Jesus name to thee." When I would find Mike on his knees like that in prayer, I knew God was listening to him and we would be just fine. He prayed us out of many messes, and he taught me how to drop to my knees in my bedroom and pray for our family when the need arose. Mike truly loved God and knew how to talk to Him.

Looking back, I realize that Mike was praying for more that just the "crisis of the moment." He stated many, many times over the years that he would "fight for our family." I believe he sent up prayers for us that he knew we needed even before we knew we needed them. There were times when the children were sick and times we did not have enough money for things we needed and God always came through for us. I sincerely believe Mike's prayers helped.

His favorite scripture was "Honor your father and mother"

(Exodus 20:12). Of course, he said it like this: "honor your fadder and mudder." Mike did. He respected us far more than "normal" children do. He knew that God meant what he said. The rest of that verse promises a longer life if we obey our parents. That could explain why Mike lived to be fifty-five years old with Down's syndrome. Maybe that is why his prayers were answered, because he believed God's promises were real.

Mike had another favorite scripture. We did not realize it was a scripture until after he was gone. He would often say, "Like mother, like daughter." He always said it after we fixed him a meal and gave him a plate of dessert. He loved my grandmother's and my mother's cooking and would say, "Mmmm, that good; you a good cook just like your mother, like mother like daughter." A month after Mike passed away my mom leaned up to me in church and handed me a note; it read, "Mike quotes scripture: Ezekiel 16:44b." I, of course, opened my Bible and looked up the scripture, which read, "Everyone who quotes proverbs will quote this proverb about you: 'Like mother, like daughter.' " I laughed inside because not only had Mike quoted scripture, but I faithfully read a chapter of proverbs every morning. Mike had reflected more insight than many people will ever acquire.

Chapter 5

My Most Embarrassing Moment

Shortly after we started taking care of Mike I became pregnant with our third child. We were very excited, but I do not think anyone was quite as excited as Mike, especially when the ultrasound confirmed that we were having a boy. Mike was getting a brother. I always thought my prayers to have a son were being answered, but I now believe that Mike's prayers to have a brother were the ones that caused the miracle.

I became unusually large in the abdomen with this pregnancy. We found out why when our son graced the world weighing ten pounds and one ounce. Being only 5 foot 2 inches and weighing 112 pounds, I looked rather deformed carrying around a ten-pound baby. I was very proud of being pregnant and enjoyed every moment of the nine months. However, I did not allow anyone to see my pregnant bare belly. It scared *me* to look at it and I figured it would scar someone for life if they saw the enormous entity. Nonetheless, one day Brad talked me into lifting my shirt over my belly so he could take a picture. When we got the picture developed I was stunned at the photo and *thought* I hid it in my bedroom, vowing never to show it to anyone. I wasn't even going to put it in our son's baby book for fear it would destroy his visions of his loving mother. So, you can understand my absolute shock when one day I was driving down the interstate highway in Oklahoma with my sister-in-law and she asked, "Angie, do you have a picture of you with your shirt pulled up exposing your pregnant belly?" I looked at her in amazement and asked her why she would ask me such a thing. "Well," she replied, "our aunt said that her friend who goes to the Assembly of God church (the church having the largest congregation in town at the time) said that Mike had a picture of your pregnant belly and he was showing it to everyone at church." When I realized what my sister-in-law had just announced to me, I screamed a scream that could be heard in the Netherlands. You know the kind of scream they do in the movies when they hear devastating news and they are driving down the highway? That is the kind of scream I belted out.

When I returned home I went straight to Mike's Bible that he carried to church and sure enough, right next to "honor your fadder and mudder" was the photo of me showing my enormous stomach to the entire world. Everyone I have told this story bursts out laughing. I do not. I did, however, realize that Mike was just so proud of his mama having a brother for him that he wanted to show the world (at my expense).

A few weeks later when Bradley "Zeke" Douthit was born, Mike was smiling from ear to ear. "That my baby brother," he would tell everyone, "bubba Zeke." Mike was very proud of Zeke and Zeke was incredibly fond of him. I remember being little and my sister and I praying for a brother that we never got. I know how Mike felt when Zeke was born. This insight helped me forget all about the embarrassment Mike had caused a few weeks earlier with the silly photo.

Chapter 6

Our Big Vacation

A few years after Mike moved in with us I got the wild idea that we should drive to Florida, go to Disney World, and cruise over to the Bahamas. At the time, I was five months pregnant with our fourth child, and Zeke was fifteen months old. We decided to leave Zeke with my parents because he was too young. I asked my sister to go, and we loaded all our stuff in our truck with a camper shell and headed to Florida.

We were like the Beverly Hillbillies entering Beverly Hills for the first time. My husband and I had never been out of the Oklahoma/Texas area and we were enchanted with all there was to see: the palm trees, bright lights, and vast array of entertainment. Mike had a ball. He smiled the entire time we were there. He loved Disney World and hugged every Disney character we encountered. He really loved the pretty princesses. We took several pictures of him and had a blast watching him and the girls meet their favorite Disney characters. We also noticed that as we would be walking around the park, Mike would suddenly stop. We would have to turn around and say, "Come on, Mike." After this occurred several times, I noticed that when Mike would see a family taking a family photo, he would stop and stand beside the family, smile, and say "cheeeese." He ended up in several family pictures with people we had never seen before. My sister and I laughed thinking of all the people that would go home, get their pictures developed (this was before digital cameras), and ask, "Who is the retarded guy in our photo?" We both still laugh every time we think about it.

Mike loved everything about Disney World except for the fact that he was not fond of the rides. Actually, it is safe to say that he really did not like them. He never really liked getting into situations where he did not feel that he was in control of his walking or riding. Cars did not scare him but a motorcycle or four-wheeler did. When you line up for a ride at Disney World they have moving sidewalks that move you along. Mike DID NOT like them. Many times my poor sister would be stuck in line trying to persuade Mike to take the first step and get on the moving sidewalk. He would shake his head and say, "I can't, maybe next year. I can't, maybe next year." After a few minutes of persuasion he would finally step on, holding on to the railing for dear life, saying, "Help me good Lord, help me Jesus."

We had made it through the majority of the colossal park and decided to take the sky trolley back across to where we began. While we were waiting in line, my sister decided that I was taking Mike on this next ride. I agreed and smiled at Mike, who was trying to get in another family photo. When it came our turn to get on the sky trolley, Brad, Mandi, and the girls hopped on board. The conductor then announced that this trolley was full and Mike and I would have to take the next one. Their trolley took off as the next one moved into place and became available. I stepped on and said, "Come on, Mike." He stood there shaking his head no. "Come on, Mike," I persuaded. "NO way, NO WAY!" he repeated. "Pleeeease," I coaxed. "NO WAY, NO WAY, MAYBE NEXT YEAR." By now I had gotten off the trolley and was trying to maneuver his body onto it. It did not work. I tried getting on the trolley and pulling on his arm. He did not move. I looked up toward the trolley my family was floating in and saw my sister waving and grinning as if to say "paybacks are rough." I tried one more attempt to get Mike on the trolley, as the people behind the conductor and us were all running out of patience. "Mike, we can get an ice cream cone if you get on this trolley." "Well, maybe just once, okay?" he finally said. I took his arm and led him on board and to his seat. He squeezed my hand tightly and began repeating "Help me good Lord, Jesus name to thee, help me good Lord, Jesus name to thee." The other riders on the trolley stared at us and smiled. I am not sure if they were smiling at how cute Mike was or how crazy I appeared. Nevertheless, we made it across Disney World and Mike got his ice cream cone.

From Florida we took a short cruise over to the Bahamas. Mike liked the boat ride and greatly enjoyed the cruise line dinner. We took a taxi to our hotel and mapped out plans for the next few days. Our first adventure would be to the beach. The next day as we were walking to the beach, we noticed a coconut tree along the sidewalk. The girls asked their daddy to get them a coconut to bring home. Brad tried to give them a rotten one lying on the ground, but they did not fall for it and demanded a "real" one. Brad scoped out the situation and realized he probably could not climb the tree to get a coconut without totally embarrassing himself in front of his family and several tourists, so he decided to pick up a rotten coconut from the ground and throw it up in the tree and knock a "real" one down. The adventure had begun.

We all stood looking up into the sky watching Brad throw with all his might at a hanging coconut. The first try failed miserably. The second try almost made it, but not quite. The girls began cheering, "Come on, Daddy, you can do it, you're the bestest daddy ever!" With inspiration like that Brad mustered up his strength and belted a rotten coconut into the air, hit a "real" coconut, and gravity took over. The "real" coconut began to drop. I remember watching it like it was in slow motion. It rolled over and over in the air as it headed for what we thought would be the ground. We watched in startled disbelief as it landed right between Mike's two blue eyes, knocked his glasses off, tumbled down Mike's face and landed on the ground next to two clapping girls. We all held our breath. There stood Mike, still looking up into the sky as if nothing had happened. "Mike, are you okay?" we all asked. After an eternal silence, Mike muttered, "I sure am." He then began to laugh, "huh huh huh hee hee." We examined his forehead and picked up his glasses, which were miraculously not broken, and determined that Mike was perfectly fine. Mike continued to laugh. We then began to roar with laughter at what had just taken place. Nearby tourists also stood shaking their heads in disbelief that Mike was okay and that we were all amused by the crazy occurrence.

Mike was nicknamed "coconut head" for the remainder of the vacation. He laughed every time we talked about it and there were many times over the years when he would start laughing and say, "Remember that coconut falling on my head?" Then we would begin laughing about it all over again. Our vacation to Florida and the Bahamas was unforgettable. It was fun, exciting, relaxing, and filled with memories. My family knows that those memories would not have been the same had Mike not been there.

Chapter 7

Our Complete Family

Four months after we came home from Florida and the Bahamas, our fourth child was born, Mackenzie Taylor Douthit. Mike was so excited when she was born. When we brought her home from the hospital, he ran around the house with his hands raised to heaven shouting "hal-lay-lu-la, hal-lay-lu-la." He kissed her on the head and said, "She so special, Mama. She my new sister." Mackenzie grew up to love Mike very much. She loved to fix his hair, and he was very patient with her. The entire time she would be working on his hair, he would sit there smiling and then would suddenly poke her in the stomach, make a gurgling sound, and say "gotcha." She would laugh and say, "Mike, hold still, I am almost finished." He had some interesting hairdos over the years. She spiked it, curled it, straightened it, and even gave him a mullet. Not every little girl has a grown man that will sit in a chair and let her fix his hair with gel and bobby pins.

My family loves to go camping at the lake or at the creek. We have spent many, many nights in tents and camper trailers with the entire family, and yes, we always took Mike with us. He loved to sit in the shade and introduce himself to anyone who passed by. "Hi, my name Mike Douthit, I getting married," he would say and then he would hold out his hand for a friendly handshake. Very few people turned Mike down on the handshake, and they would usually congratulate him on getting married. Sadly, he never got to do it.

One night we were sitting around the campfire. Most people camping near us were already settled down for the night, and it was unusually quiet. I set my lounge chair out and as I began to sit down; the middle legs gave out, folded under the chair, and down I went on the ground with a loud thud. Mike began to laugh. He not only laughed, he slapped his knees and rocked back and forth in his lawn chair. He laughed so loud and long that we also began to laugh because he was so funny. We laughed so loud and so long that we started to wake up people camping around us. We tried to stop, but could not because Mike could not stop. After what seemed like forever, Mike stopped, so we settled down. When we finally stopped laughing, we realized that I was still sitting on the ground where I had fallen and I could not get up. Mike started laughing again and so began the whole scenario all over. When we were finally able to contain ourselves we held our hurting stomach muscles and decided that it was time to go to bed so that our neighbors could get some rest. I looked at Mike and said, "Head to bed, Fred." He replied, "Okay, Wilma." Yes, the laughter took over once again.

Our church decided to join the church summer softball league that next year. It was Brad's first time to really play any form of baseball/softball, but being the athletic guy that he is, he caught on quite fast. With Mike cheering him on, how could he be anything but wonderful? Mike loved to go to the ball games and was the loudest cheerleader in the stands. He could be heard all over the entire ballpark yelling "YAY, DADDY DARLING DEAR" or "THAT MY DADDY, YAY!!!" The cheering would not have been so bad except for the fact that Mike did not understand the concept of baseball, meaning that when you strike out, fly out, or drop the ball it is a bad thing and quite embarrassing when someone is cheering for you when you make one of those undesirable mistakes.

Brad's mom made the mistake of telling Mike that his uncle called him Lambie Pie when he was young and that was his nickname. Mike quickly picked it up and used it in the most uncomfortable moments. Brad would put his head down and shake it back and forth when he would fly out and Mike would stand up in the bleachers and begin his chorus of "YAY, Lambie Pie!" The people in the stands would look at us, shake their heads, and chuckle.

One game, our church played against the church Mike grew up in, the First Assembly of God church. Mike loved both churches, so it was hard for him to decide whom to cheer for. Mike, being the lovable guy he was, cheered for both teams. He would stand up, raise his plump arms in the air, and shout, "Yay, I'm a baptacostal." It amazed me that Mike knew to take the words Baptist and Pentecostal, and put them together to form a new word. We all laughed and knew exactly what he was talking about.

The trend continued when our children started playing sports, Mike would yell, "YAY, ZEKE, THAT MY BROTHER AND I LOVE HIM, THANK YOU JESUS FOR MY DARLING BROTHER." Zeke would just smile and wave at him in the stands. The girls would get a little embarrassed when they were young, but as they got older and were cheerleaders, they would wave to the stands and say, "Hey, Mike." Then they would look at their friends and say, "That's my brother Mike." Before long several girls and boys would be saying hello to Mike as we would enter the football stadium. Many of them would sit next to him and chat. He always insisted on sitting in the first row because climbing stairs was not to his liking. He was also able to shake everyone's hand as they walked by and say, "Hi, I'm Mike Douthit and I'm getting married." Most responded with a smile, a handshake, and the reply, "That's nice, Mike."

I did not realize what an entrance we made walking into those ballgames until Mike passed away and many people, some of whom I did not even know, would walk up to me and say, "I am so sorry about Mike; I would see you all at the ballgames together." It's going to be very tough and different this first year when Zeke plays football and the girls cheer and Mike is not with us.

Chapter 8

Mike's Jc

Mike got a job. The Volunteers of America did us a favor and found Mike a job and a job coach who would go with Mike to his work. The coach would help train him and make sure he was not doing anything incorrectly. Eventually, when the job coaches felt sure the worker was trustworthy, they would leave them for a few hours on the job to work independently.

Mike's job was to clean and dust in a local furniture store. He cleaned the bathrooms and dusted the furniture. He loved working and enjoyed meeting new people so he could tell them that he was getting married and was pregnant. By the way, I had just about had Mike convinced that a man could not have a baby when we turned on the TV and there stood Arnold Schwarzenegger nine months pregnant about to give birth. Mike stared at the television and said, "See, Mama, men can have babies." It is hard to argue with anything Arnie can do. Anyway, Mike had proved himself worthy to be left alone on the job (but not for long).

A few days after his promotion, I went in the furniture store to pick up Mike from work. An angry store manager met me at the door and explained that Mike was not welcome to come back. "You are firing Mike?" I asked. "Yes!" explained the red-faced manager. "He switched a few tags on some chairs, and I was forced to sell

sive chairs at a ridiculously low price." "Oh!" I replied, trying
t to giggle. I was getting ready to apologize but the man kept
complaining about Mike. Suddenly the mother hen in me kicked
in and I turned to the defense and told the irritated man that Mike
did not understand what he had done. I then told Mike to come
with me because we were leaving. When we were in the car, I asked
Mike why he had changed the prices on the chairs and he replied,
"They were too expensive." It made perfect sense to me.

For years when we would drive past that furniture store Mike
would say, "That man fired me, Mama, over those price tags on the
chairs." "He sure did," I would say, "but some lucky customer got
blessed that day because you priced those chairs as they should have
been, Mike." "I sure did," he would always say.

Chapter 9

Becky

The women working for Volunteers of America were wonderful. Since the job idea did not work out for Mike, they felt sorry for him and asked if he could go bowling with them. I said he could, and they showed up the next day to get him. When they entered, they had a client with them named Becky. She was funny and quickly became friends with Mike. They had a blast together laughing and telling jokes only they understood. They loved bowling, eating, and going to dances. Mike greatly enjoyed going places with the volunteers and Becky.

Mike loved Becky. It was during this time that Mike began saying he was getting married to Becky. He became obsessed with the idea. One afternoon, on mine and Brad's wedding anniversary, Mike came out of his bedroom dressed in his three-piece suit with a tie and his hair slicked over to the side. "What are you doing, Mike?" I asked. He grinned, batted his eyelashes, and announced "I getting married today on your anniversary. We share an anniversary, okay?" I chuckled and explained to him that Becky probably wasn't ready for it today. He simply said, "Maybe next year, okay?" "Maybe next year," I replied.

A few years after Mike met Becky, her family moved her to a nice group home in a town about forty minutes away. Mike visited her a few times and went with her to a Halloween party dressed as Batman, but then never got to see her again. In spite of that, until the day he went into a coma, he still told EVERYONE he talked to that he was marrying Becky. Even in the hospital with a broken leg, he told every doctor and nurse that he was getting married to Becky.

Mike never got to marry Becky. However, he would have made a wonderful husband. He would have loved her unconditionally. He would have never had an affair. He would have never loved money or hobbies more than her. He would have put God first in their marriage and prayed for her daily. He would have told her she was beautiful and that he loved her everyday. He would have made her laugh when times were tough. And, he would have never complained about her cooking. In my eyes, he would have been the perfect husband.

Chapter 10

The Day Care

When our children were little, I wanted to be a stay-at-home mom. I loved being home with the kids and Mike, but of course we needed extra income. I decided to open a small day care in our home. It was perfect at the time. I was home caring for my own children, so why not share my time with other children. For six years I took care of five to seven other children and loved every minute of it. Mike also loved all the kids, and the kids loved him just as much.

Children are different from adults. Children were not afraid of Mike. They knew he was different, but they adored him. We could be at Wal-Mart and children would begin to talk to Mike. Many times their parents would take their children by the hand and lead them away from us. I would just shake my head and think of the joy those parents were denying their children. I only had one parent not feel comfortable bringing their child to our day care because of Mike. The rest loved him and enjoyed talking to him. Mike was a wonderful help with the kids. He could stand near the swing set and push children for hours on the swings. He never seemed to tire of playing with them.

Some of the best times during the day care days were Mike's birthdays. "December 16, 1952," he would say, "that my birthday." So, every December 16 we would buy party hats, balloons, and a chocolate cake with candles, set all the children around the table, and sing "Happy Birthday" to Mike. He would grin from ear to ear, make a wish, and blow out his candles. The children ate cake and ice cream with him and laughed at his chocolate lips. He would then open his presents. No matter what he opened, he would say, "Woo-wee, look, Mama, that's nice, isn't that pretty?" and he would hold it up to his face and smile for a picture. After several years Brad began to say, "Mike, we could wrap up dog poop and you would say, 'Isn't that nice.' " Mike would laugh and say, "I love you, Daddy darling dear." "I love you too, Mike," would always be Brad's laughing response.

Every day at 1:00 would be "nap time" for the day care. Every child would lay down at 1:00 and go to sleep until 3:15, when we would have to go pick up the school-age children from school. I started noticing that every day at 1:00 when I would say "nap time," Mike would walk to his room, lie down, and go to sleep. That was one of the really great things about Mike; he was just as much a child as he was an adult.

When our youngest child Mackenzie entered first grade, I knew it was time for me to close the day care, finish my college degree, and follow my dream of becoming a schoolteacher. (Mike thought that was cool because his biological mother had also been a school-teacher.) Closing the day care was very sad and bittersweet because the seven little boys I had been watching for quite a while and their mothers were precious. I hated telling them my plans but knew it was for the best. Mike hated seeing the boys leave for the last time and even cried when they left. I was sad because I would miss the boys and their mothers, but I was also terrified because of the money we would be losing. Mike, sensing my frustration and pain, put his hand on my shoulder and said, "It be okay, Mama; you'll see time comes." I knew he was correct once again.

Chapter 11

Back to Work

When I started back to college I realized that I needed a place for Mike to stay. My grandparents volunteered, and Mike was overjoyed because he *loved* Grandma's cooking. She had a special seat for him in her dining area and he knew it was his chair. I would drop him off in the mornings and he would head straight for his chair and inquire where breakfast was. Mike also loved to give my grandfather a hard time. They made it a daily habit of teasing each other. Grandpa would pretend to take Mike's plate of dinner away and Mike would say to him, "Watch it, mister," and the game would continue until Mike would pretend to stab Grandpa with his fork.

He loved going to my grandparents' home. He would say, "Monday, Wednesday, Friday I go to Grandma's." And then he would ask every morning, "Is it Monday, Wednesday, Friday?" On the days I would say "No, Mike, you stay home with me today," he would lower his head and say, "The nice old people miss me today." "Yes, they will Mike," I admitted. Then he would exhale very loudly to let me know he was not happy about staying home with me. It was the cooking. Cooking is not one of my gifts. My paternal grandmother was an expert in the kitchen. Both my maternal grandma and my mother are excellent cooks, but that gene jumped right over me and landed on two of my daughters (thankfully). My daughter

Whitney looked at me one day and said, "It's okay, Mom, you make wonderful frozen food; you are the Frozen Food Queen." "Thanks, maybe someday I will write a cookbook on how to make great frozen food," I laughed.

Mike continued to stay at my grandparents' house three days a week while I finished college and then remained on that schedule after I landed a teaching job. My mom started keeping him on Tuesday and Thursday. He loved it and would complain during summer, spring, and Christmas breaks when he could not go to their houses. I knew he still loved me and was very pleased that he enjoyed going to their homes so much. It took a huge worry off of my shoulders to know he was well cared for during the day. I am also glad that my mom and grandparents got to spend quality time with Mike during his last seven years on this earth.

I will never forget one particular afternoon I picked up Mike from my mom's. We got in the van, and I asked him how his day went. He responded by shaking his head and saying, "Grandma Jayne is mad; she went off like a Roman candle." After several moments of laughter on my part, I asked him why she was so mad. "I don't know; she needs Jesus today," he replied. "I'm sure she does," I said. "Lord help her," he replied, and I roared with laughter once again. After that day, every time I would pick him up from Mom's I would ask him if Grandma Jayne went off like a Roman candle today and he would slap his knee, laugh, and say "She sure did."

I teach third grade, and I loved to bring Mike to my class for the students to meet him. He would walk in, smile, wave his fingers, tilt his head to the side, and say, "Hi, how are you? I getting married tomorrow."

He kept the kids spellbound. They would ask him questions and laugh at his adorable responses. It was great for the students to see that a person with Down's syndrome could be harmless, kind, and loving. My students asked about him often and loved for me to tell them a "Mike story." If they were good, as a reward, I would try to tell them one at the end of the day. My youngest daughter asked if she could take Mike to show-and-tell at her school. Brad and I laughed at her innocence, but realized how proud of him she was. We then discussed how proud of him all of us were. We loved him and wanted everyone to see how incredible he was.

Chapter 12

Everyone Loves Mike

Everyone seemed to like Mike. We would be in a town thirty miles away, shopping at the mall, and people would stop and say, "Hi Mike, how are you doing?" He would respond by saying "My name Mike Douthit, I getting adopted by Mr. and Mrs. Brad Douthit, and I getting married tomorrow." They would hug him and say, "It sure is good to see you, Mike."

Mike tried to hug everyone. I worked relentlessly to get him to shake hands with people but he always wanted to hug them. Especially pretty women. He used to tell me that I looked just like Farrah Fawcett. Mom would hear him tell me that, so one day she decided to ask Mike whom he thought she looked like. She said, "Mike, who do I look like?" He grinned and without hesitation he replied, "Barbara Bush." Mom made a disgusted face because Barbara is much older than her, but the rest of us in the family rolled on the floor with laughter. Mike thought it was quite a compliment. To him, Barbara Bush was beautiful because she was a Republican and he was a die-hard Republican. He walked over, hugged Mom, and told her she was beautiful.

With Mike being such a people person it truly surprised me one day when the doorbell rang and a mad neighbor lady and her bewildered daughter stood at my door ranting and raving and using

35

language only heard on Comedy Central Roasts. I asked her what was wrong and soon discovered that she was furious with Mike. With surprise on my face and in my voice, I asked her what in the world he could have done to make her so angry. She explained in her interesting language that Mike had opened her door and put her newspaper on her entry floor. She then went on to demand that he never come in her house again. Still not understanding why she was so enraged, I promised her that he would never enter her house again and tried to explain that he thought he was doing her a favor by taking her newspaper to her. She continued to rant and rave and I firmly had to tell her to leave and to never come to our house acting and talking like that ever again. When she left I talked to Mike about not entering people's houses and how some people are not as friendly and kind as others. He put his hand on my shoulder and simply said, "She needs Jesus." I agreed with him wholeheartedly.

Mike was a teenager when his mother built the home that we shared with him. Some current neighbors lived in the neighborhood when Mike and his mother moved in. They have told me many funny stories about Mike. I often wonder what they think of us caring for Mike compared to when his mother cared for him. I am sure they have stood in awe at the many strange things we have done, but over the years they have thanked us for taking such good care of him.

Mike loved to walk around the block and say "hello" to the neighbors. One day I loaded all of the day care children into my van to go pick up the schoolchildren. Mike came walking around the corner, so I waved and told him to come and get in the van. When I looked to my left, I realized that every neighbor's trash dumpster was out in the middle of the road. I looked at Mike and he grinned and said, "Today's trash day, Mama." I responded with, "And, did you push all of these nice people's trash dumpsters into the middle of the road?" "I sure did," he proudly replied. "Mike, what am I going to do with you?" I asked, and then began driving around the block, stopping every 20 feet to push a trash dumpster back to the curb before the trash man showed up and the nice neighbors became aggravated. Every time I got back in the van to drive to the next dumpster Mike would say, "You so nice, Mama, I love you." "I love you too, Mike, but please don't ever do this again, okay?" "Okay, Mama."

One day when I went to pick up the kids, Mike stayed behind to walk around the block. When I got home there was a note on the door stating that I owed $15 for address numbers being painted on the curb. I looked at Mike. He smiled and said, "He a nice man, Mama." "Mike, did you tell this man to paint numbers on our curb?" "I sure did." He smiled from ear to ear. I looked down the road and one of my neighbor friends came walking to my house, laughing. She told me that the same man came to her house asking to paint numbers on her curb and he told her that he had painted them on mine. She asked him who told him to since she noticed that my van was gone. He pointed at Mike, who was standing in the driveway blowing big kisses at people driving by. My neighbor said she looked at the strange man and said, "Mike? He thinks he's pregnant, you shouldn't listen to him." The man just shook his head and left. We never saw the man again.

Mike loved to embarrass me. I am still not sure if he did it on purpose or not, but his fun-loving heart just couldn't help it sometimes. One day I was driving down the interstate with Mike sitting in his passenger side backseat. I began to notice that several truckers were honking and waving at me. I waved at the first few but started to become leery when they kept honking. I checked to make sure my shirt was buttoned properly and then turned my head to discover that Mike was using his sign language once again to get the truckers to honk at us. They weren't waving at me at all; they were waving and honking at Mike. He was laughing and grinning with his crooked, one-of-a-kind smile.

Another day we were sitting in the waiting room at the doctor's office when a large woman walked in and signed her name on the patient list. Mike looked at her and then at me and said very loudly, "She needs to lose weight just like me, Mama." The entire waiting room heard him and I tried to play it off by saying "No, Mike, she is just right." "No, she look like me, she's overweight, too." Honestly, what can you say at a moment like that? I just put my head down and tried to finish reading my magazine, pretending that the entire waiting room was not staring at us and giggling.

On another occasion we were at the mall and a rather sizeable woman walked by and he said at full volume, "Look Mama, she pregnant like me," and smiled at the woman as he patted his overgrown belly. She did not smile back. She was not pregnant. Mike could not understand why she did not act like she was happy. I tried to explain to him that most people do not like being chubby, even though he did. He hated to be told that he was losing weight. He would become irritated with you and say, "No, I'm not. I was born chubby and I be overweight all my life." I would shake my head and marvel at all the weight-loss programs in America for people trying to lose weight, and Mike thought being overweight was a blessing.

Another of our most embarrassing moments was at Wal-Mart during the Christmas season. I had taken Mike to Wal-Mart so that he could shop for his brother and sisters. I was in a bit of a hurry and walking fast through the crazy crowd of Christmas shoppers when I heard, "Mama." I turned around and gasped in shock as I saw Mike standing there right next to the perfume aisle with his jeans fallen down to his ankles.

He had forgotten to put his belt on. I saw people walking way around Mike with his whitie tighties showing for the whole store to see. I immediately ran to him, faced him, bent over to pick up his pants, and began to pull them up. People were really looking at us strangely now, and walking way around us as we were still in the middle of the aisle. I was facing him with my arms around him as

I shimmied his pants up and tucked his shirt in. I looked up to see that we were standing right under a security camera. We both smiled and waved at the camera. I pictured security guards and managers staring at the strange lady pulling up the pants of the funny-looking, older man. Once again I laughed and thought of what a fun sense of humor God must have.

Chapter 13

Mike the Republican

Mike was a strong Republican. So much so that one year on his birthday I asked him if he wanted to play Pin the Tale on the Donkey. He replied by saying that he would only play Pin the Tale on the Elephant because the Republican's symbol was an elephant.

Mike knew all of the president's names, what their initials stood for, and their first ladies' names. He could also tell you which ones were Democrats and which ones were Republicans. I was told that his entire family were registered Democrats. Somewhere down the road, Mike decided to become a Republican.

Every election year I took Mike to vote. He knew exactly whom he wanted to vote for. I just had to help him mark the lines correctly. I will never forget the last presidential election he got to vote in. We live in a county that is considered to be a democratic county, but Mike was a huge George W. Bush fan. We walked in to find the line to vote very long, stretching all the way to the back door. When we entered I noticed how quiet it was and tried to whisper when I talked to Mike. Suddenly in the awkward silence, Mike raised both hands in the air and yelled in his scruffy voice: "YAY, Republicans are winning, YAY George Bush!" Everyone turned to stare at us. The looks we received that evening were priceless. In Mike's innocence he told the entire county whom he was voting for.

Chapter 14

"Go Shave, Mike!"

Mike shaved his face with a cordless razor. He usually did a good job except for the occasional times when he would shave his sideburns up to the side of his head. Every morning I would say "Go shave, Mike," and he would head to his bathroom. One day he went into his room and came out clearly not having shaven. I kept telling him to go shave, and he would leave and come back unshaven. Finally, I began to inquire why he was not shaving. The conversation went something like this.

"Mike, why won't you shave?"

"I don't have my razor."

"Where is it?"

"I buried it."

"You buried it?"

"Yes, I sure did."

"Where did you bury your razor, Mike?"

"Outside."

"Why did you bury your razor?" (This is the good part.)

"The battery was DEAD."

"You buried your razor because the battery was dead?"

"Yes, Mama, I sure did."

After I stopped laughing and realized why he had buried the

43

razor, I asked if he could go show Kaylee where he had buried it. Kaylee followed Mike outside to the side of the house and returned within minutes carrying a muddy cordless razor. We cleaned it up, charged the battery, and laughed while Mike shaved.

If I had a dollar for every time I told him to go shave, I would be a wealthy lady. It became the joke of the house. When the kids' friends would walk in they would say, "Go shave, Mike." He would laugh and say, "You so funny." After Mike passed away, I cleaned his room and bathroom. I thought I had packed everything and asked his cousin to come and see if she wanted some of his items. We walked into his bathroom and there on his sink lay his cordless razor. I instantly teared up and had to walk out of the room as I remembered all of the times I had to tell Mike to go shave and the time he buried his razor because the battery was dead.

Chapter 15

The Dentist's Office

When my children were little, the dentist decided that I needed my wisdom teeth extracted. I found a sitter and asked Mom to take me to the dentist since they would be putting me to sleep for the procedure. For reasons I cannot recall, we took Mike with us. The dentist's office had an unusually large waiting room, and I remember it being very full of waiting patients. I was soon called in to surgery as the nurses explained that my mother could come in with me during the end of my recovery and could help me to the car.

I do not remember very much about the procedure, as I am one of those people who become quite loopy when given any kind of medication. What I do remember is still etched in my memory and I cackle every time I picture it in my head.

Mom had left Mike in the waiting room with strict instructions to stay put and not to bother the nice people sitting near him. Mike agreed and Mom went back to aid her swollen-jawed daughter. I finally recovered from the anesthetic and my mother helped me walk back to the waiting room.

When we entered the waiting room, there on his knees facing his chair with his hands folded in prayer and his eyes looking toward heaven, Mike was praying aloud for his "mama." "Dear Jesus, help my mama, keep her safe and help her, Jesus name to Thee." He was repeating this phrase over and over. The entire audience in the crowded waiting room had their eyes fixed on Mike and could not wait to see who "mama" was.

I cannot describe the looks on their faces when they discovered that "mama" was in her twenties while this man on his knees was obviously in his mid forties. I walked over to Mike and helped him up from his knees. He grabbed me and hugged me tight. "You okay, Mama?" he asked. "I am just fine, Mikey, lets go home," was my reply. We walked out of the clinic, sat in the car, and laughed until our sides hurt. Mike could make even dental surgery funny.

We received many strange looks over the years from people in Wal-Mart and the grocery store when Mike would call me "mama" and Brad "daddy." We would just smile and silently thank the good Lord for allowing us the blessing of living with Mike.

Chapter 16

Mike's Fears

When we first started caring for Mike, he loved to swim. He would get in the pool, walk around, put his face in the water, and blow bubbles. Brad and I would take him to our city pool and he would entertain the kids with his fish noises and bubble blowing. But as he got older he became afraid of the water. On the Fourth of July, our city swimming pool has a free day. The entire town comes out to swim. On this particular holiday, we went to join the fun.

I asked Mike if he wanted to get in the water and he said yes. I helped lower him into the end of the pool where it began with three feet of water. He was having a blast blowing bubbles at the kids and splashing me. As long as he was close enough to touch the side of the pool he was fine.

We had been swimming about thirty minutes when the lifeguards blew their whistles for all of us to get out for break time. I got the kids out and began trying to get Mike out. I tried pushing him up. I tried pulling him out. I tried rolling him out. Nothing was working. You are probably asking yourself right now, "Why didn't she just use the ladder?" Well, that was my next resort but the ladder was located in five feet of water. I am only five foot two inches and Mike is only five foot five inches, so I had to walk Mike down into water that was almost over our heads.

I slowly began the menial task. We bounced down the side of the pool to the ladder. When we got there Mike refused to climb up. I tried pushing, pulling, hoisting, but nothing worked. Every time I tried to push or pull, he would hug me and say "I love you, Mama darling." I would respond with, "I love you, too, but we have to get out of this pool before we get into trouble." As you can guess, by then we had a rather large crowd watching us to see how I was going to get this Down's syndrome man out of the pool in five feet of water. One of the lifeguards noticed us and *finally* offered to help.

Mike, of course, did not trust the lifeguard and would not let him pull him up. However, they informed me that they did have a hydraulic lift with a chair for handicapped people. They lowered it into the water and I helped Mike sit in the chair. I buckled him in but he immediately grabbed hold of the metal pole that held the chair. He did not just grab it, he bear-hugged it and would not let go. They could not lift the hydraulic chair up until Mike let go of the pole. I tried to convince him to let go but he just shook his head back and forth saying, "I scared, Mama, I scared."

After what seemed like eternity, I finally convinced him to let go of the pole and take hold of my hand so they could lift him out of the water. By now every swimmer at the pool was gathered around to see the scared retarded man being lifted out of the pool. They slowly lifted him up, we unbuckled him and stood him up, and he raised both his arms like a boxer taking his victory lap around the ring and shouted, "Yeah, I did it! I did it, Mama!" Immediately, the whistle blew and the voice over the speaker said, "Back in the pool, swimmers; the break is over, it's time to swim." The exhausted lifeguard looked at me and we both burst into laughter. That was the last time Mike let me put him in a pool. When we would ask him to swim he would smile and say, "No thank you, maybe next year."

Mike had not only a fear of water, but also a crazy fear of escalators and carnival rides. One weekend we were at the airport to pick up my sister. We headed for the escalator to go downstairs. When Mike saw the moving stairs, he backed up and began saying, "No thank you, no thank you." I said, "Come on, Mike, it will be fun."

"No way, NO WAY," he began to say louder and louder. I felt like Tom Cruise in *Rain Man*. He was clearly not getting on the escalator. We had to turn around and walk several yards to find an elevator to get Mike to the first floor.

When we returned home I told Brad the story of Mike and his refusal to get on the escalator, and he claimed that he could have talked Mike into getting on the escalator. "Whatever! He will never get on an escalator," I insisted. A few weeks later we were visiting my sister at college and decided to go to the mall. It just happened to be around Christmas time, and the mall, of course, was full of shoppers. We entered JC Penney, and lo and behold, they had an escalator. Brad's eyes widened and he said, "Come on Mike, we are going for a ride." We walked toward the escalator, and Mike began saying, "No thank you, no thank you," and "No way, no way." But, Mike loved his daddy and allowed Brad to put him on that moving escalator. We stood in amazement as we watched him and Brad rise to the next floor with Mike smiling, holding on to Brad's arm and waving to the crowd the entire way up. We all jumped on and headed up behind them. When we reached the top, Brad was smiling and saying, "See, I told you I could get him to ride it." We congratulated him and told Mike how proud of him we were until … we began to smell what would become known as the "Mike Smell."

In the excitement of finally getting on an escalator, Mike had messed his drawers. "What are we going to do?" Brad asked. "WE are going to stand out here and wait while YOU take Mike in the bathroom and help him remove his underwear and throw them in the trash can. You will then help him clean his bottom." Brad looked around at me and the kids, my sister and her college friends, my parents, and then at Mike. He dropped his head, took Mike by the hand, and headed for the bathroom. Mike turned around and blew kisses to us. We chuckled at this strange event occurring in the mall. We waited outside the restroom and within a few minutes two young boys came running out giggling and fanning their noses. We just stood there and laughed.

Brad and Mike finally came slowly out of the bathroom. "Never again," was all Brad would say. Mike chimed in with "I love you, Daddy darling dear." We gave Mike high fives as he winked at us. Mike never got on an escalator again.

Chapter 17

"Give It to Mike, He'll Eat Anything"

One year for New Year's Eve we decided to have a nice, quiet, sit-down dinner at my mother's; complete with the "good dishes" and Dad's famous fondue. We were very excited about this nice dinner. Mom had prepared for it all day, and the table looked magnificent. We had salad, baked potatoes, homemade bread, cranberry sauce, iced tea, and steak and shrimp to be cooked in the fondue pots. Mike was sitting between Whitney and my dad, rubbing his tummy saying, "Mmmmm, this looks good, Grandma." I cooked his steak and shrimp for him in the fondue pot so he would not burn himself, and he was absolutely enjoying every minute of this meal.

Eating was his favorite thing to do. He loved to eat more than anyone I have ever met. I used to say he did not have a shut-off valve. I honestly believe he was unaware when he was full. He could eat forever. One time we wanted to see how much he could actually eat before he got full. He ate and ate and ate until *I* could not take it anymore. Worried that he was going to truly explode, I made him stop. He just smiled, looked at Brad, and whispered, "We have dessert now?" He was truly a bottomless pit.

I worked very hard with him so he would be a clean eater and not eat with his mouth open. People who live with Down's syndrome have an extra-thick tongue and it is hard for them to keep their mouths closed sometimes. I believe Mike's real mother had taught him to be a neat eater, but there were times when he was trying to eat fast and he would get a little messy. At those times I would say, "Mike, eat with your mouth closed, please." He would squeeze both lips together and make a kissing face like a fish and chew. His fish lips would move up and down until he swallowed. It was quite humorous. It was one of those faces only a mother could love. I thought it was adorable.

Back to the holiday celebration. Mike was trying his best to use his manners at the table. We were well into the meal, with our plates filled and the fondue pots cooking feverishly. All of a sudden, from out of nowhere, without any warning, Mike sneezed. Now, Mike did not sneeze like most humans. When he sneezed his hand never quite made it to his mouth and nose in time to stop any droplets from flying straight ahead. This sneeze was no different. He sneezed and, as if in slow motion, clear liquid (we are still not sure if the liquid came from his mouth or his nose) came flying out and landed on Whitney's plate on top of a piece of freshly cooked shrimp. In that unforgettable split second everyone at the table, sixteen of us to be exact, gasped and made the same grossed out face. Whitney looked mortified and my dad turned his head away from the shrimp and began to repeat, "Get it out of here; throw it away, just get it out of here and throw it away." At the same time my mother, who can't stand to waste any food no matter what the situation, began to say, "Oh, Whitney, just wash it off in the sink, it will be fine. I promise, it will be okay, just go wash it off."

Poor Whitney sat there looking at her plate, not knowing what to do. Everyone began shouting his or her opinions of whom she should listen to. In the middle of the chaos I looked at Mike, who was happily eating his New Year's Eve dinner and grinning. He was happy as a lark. Whitney finally picked up her sneeze-infested shrimp and threw it away. I glanced around the room and made eye contact with Kaylee and my sister and we lost it. We laughed until our sides ached.

For several years after this unforgettable episode, my children would have friends over and they would bring them into the kitchen and say, "Hey Mom, tell my friends about Mike sneezing on Whitney's shrimp." Their friends were always amused and thought it was pretty cool. Mike would join in the laughter and hug whoever was standing nearby.

Chapter 18

My Goofy Family

As the kids got older, they helped me care for Mike. One day I realized how strange life was. When the kids were little, Mike had helped me take care of them. Now that he was aging and they were teenagers, they helped me take care of him.

I had left him with Kaylee one afternoon with instructions for her to fix Mike a sandwich, chips, and a drink. Mike did not like to eat a sandwich without chips and he never wanted a hamburger without french fries and a Coke. When we would pull into McDonalds, he would simply say "hamburger, french fries, and Coke, please." So Kaylee knew to give him the works.

I came home about an hour later and found Mike sitting at the table with an empty plate in front of him with two red bologna rings lying on the side. I looked at him and he smiled. Kaylee came walking around the corner and I asked her about the bologna rings. She looked at Mike and asked, "What's wrong? Don't you like the rings?"

"Of course he doesn't like them, Kaylee," I responded.

"Why not?" she asked with a puzzled look on her face.

"Because they taste bad and you are not supposed to eat them."

"You're not? I always do," she replied. I stood there and looked at my teenage daughter in amused disbelief and dared to ask, "Are you telling me that you always eat the ring around the bologna?"

"Yes, aren't you supposed to?"

I began to laugh. "Kaylee," I began, "obviously even Mike knows to take the bologna rings off of the sandwich you made him."

Mike then began to laugh and slap his knee. He said, "HEE HEE HEE Mama, you have two retardeds in this family." I responded with, "I know, Mike, I have a lot of retardeds in this family."

Not only did my own children love Mike, so did our extended families. Both Brad's and my family adored him. It did not matter which side of the family was having the family reunion, everyone there would hug Mike and offer him some more dessert. He also adored all of them, and we had seventeen years of wonderful, memorable, Thanksgiving and Christmas celebrations with Mike. He loved teasing them and rejoiced every time someone in the family gave birth to a precious new baby. "I have a new cousin," he would announce, and he would remember their middle names and their birth weight. He loved how many aunts and uncles he had and always made sure each one said hello to him and gave him a hug before we left.

My cousin Sam adored Mike. When Sam was in college he would come and get Mike and take him to play Frisbee Golf. I was amazed at a college kid wanting to spend time with a man with Down's syndrome. Sam would even take Mike places with him and his girlfriend. Sam later became a preacher. Mike loved to hear him preach. Mike also loved Sam's dad, who was also a preacher. Uncle Robert teased Mike at every family dinner and Mike growled at him. They were both wonderful with Mike and I am thankful for their kindness to him.

I realized after we lost Mike just how much he had meant to our extended family. They all sobbed as they heard of his death, and their love and support were astounding during the funeral and the months that followed.

Chapter 19

Down's Syndrome

Mike could recognize other people afflicted with Down's syndrome. He would see a person with Down's syndrome when were out somewhere, and he would say, "Look, Mama, he/she look like me." Sure enough, every time he said that I would turn around and see a person with Down's syndrome.

One day at Wal-Mart we met a mother who I will never forget. I was walking down a food aisle when I realized Mike was not right with me. I turned around and found Mike bent over talking to a small child in a shopping cart. He looked at me and said once again, "Look, Mama, he look like me." I smiled at this adorable little boy who was grinning at Mike as Mike played with the child's hands. I looked at the mother and watched as tears filled her eyes as she observed the situation in front of her. I introduced Mike and myself, and explained to her that Mike was fifty years old. He looked at her and said, "I born December 16, 1952." Then he looked back toward the boy and began talking to him. I felt led to tell the mother about Mike and how healthy he was for a person with Down's syndrome. We both agreed how wonderful and amazing people who live with Down's syndrome are. She swallowed back tears as she told of her son's many ailments. "His name is Camden," she stated. "We don't know how long he will live, but it is encouraging to meet someone like Mike who overcame his handicaps and who is so happy." I told her that Mike was always in a good mood. Mike hugged both of them bye and blew a kiss to Camden as we walked away.

A year and a half later, Mike and I were at Wal-Mart. We came around a corner into another aisle and a woman stopped us and said, "Mike, I have been coming to Wal-Mart for months hoping to run into you two. I am Camden's mother." I remembered who she was and asked her how Camden was doing. She looked me in the eyes and with a sad voice she slowly whispered, "We lost Camden six months ago. I never forgot Mike and how inspiring he was, and I have been looking for you so I could give him something." She reached into her purse and brought out a photo of Camden. She handed it to Mike and he took it and smiled. He then must have sensed her sadness because he reached out his chubby short arms and hugged her and kissed her on the cheek. She told him he was an incredible person. He looked her in the eyes and said, "I will pray for you." And then we parted ways. On the back of the picture it said, "To Mike, from Camden."

I think of her sometimes and wish I had had a picture of Mike to give her. At that moment I realized what a special, amazing person I was caring for and living with. Mike truly did have a special link with God.

Chapter 20

Funny Mike

Mike loved to save newspaper clippings and had quite a collection from over the years. One day he came out of his room and said, "Look Mama, this is Aunt Rhonda," as he handed me a newspaper clipping. I looked at the photo in disbelief. It was a picture of one of my best friends with one of her babies that she had before I had even known her. I read the article, then called my friend and asked her about it. She said that she was in the newspaper with her new baby but it was before she knew our family and Mike. We never discovered why he had clipped the article and how it happened to be my good friend Rhonda. We did talk of the incident often and laughed about how inquisitive Mike was.

Whitney's high school history teacher grew up with Mike, having attended the First Assembly of God church with him. He loved to tell her stories about Mike when he was younger. He said that when he was a teenager he was in the men's restroom at church, standing at the urinal, when suddenly out from under the stall next to him came a hand that grabbed his ankle and a voice that said, "Gotcha!" The voice then began to laugh hysterically and he knew it was Mike. Only Mike could get away with doing something like that and have all of us think it was funny.

He also told us of a time when Mike had found his mother's

church directory and called every phone number to invite people to his wedding shower. Several members showed up with gifts the next Sunday. His mother was embarrassed and explained to the congregation that he was not getting married.

Mike's pastor's son told us about growing up with Mike. He explained that when they were teenagers, Mike became concerned about his grandparents' sick dog, Lassie. He was so worried about Lassie being ill that he called 911 and directed the ambulance drivers to the rural farm his grandparents lived on. The 911 dispatcher thought Mike had said, "*Leslie* is sick and needs an ambulance." When the paramedics arrived and found a sick collie dog named Lassie, they were not happy. Mike's mother had to explain to the hospital that Mike was only trying to help.

One weekend we were at Lake Eufaula with my parents and sister's family for a mini-vacation. We stayed in a one-room cabin with wall-to-wall beds. We had just gotten situated for the night and thought we had the kids asleep, when suddenly piercing the silence was Mike's ghostly voice calling, "WOOOOOOOOOOO, WOOOOOOOOO!" He sounded just like the scary sounds you hear at Halloween spook houses. We calmed down the children and lay silently once more, until Mike sounded again, "WOOOOOOO, WOOOOOOO!" Hysterical laughter took over. We laughed for over an hour as each one of us made goofy sounds into the quiet cabin. To this day when we go to Lake Eufaula, my kids wait until bedtime and then begin their "Mike sounds."

Chapter 21

The Baseball Game

It became more and more difficult for Mike to get in and out of cars and to climb up and down steps as he began to age. That never stopped us though. One of us would take one arm and another would take the other arm, and we would walk Mike wherever we needed to go. Dad, Mom, Brad, the kids, and I took Mike to a baseball game in Kansas City one steamy, hot July. We had wonderful seats down close to the field. We were all excited about our great seats, not thinking how many steps we had to walk down to get to our destination. Everyone took off quickly to their seats. Everyone that is, except Mike and me. We painfully walked down every step carefully and slowly with me holding his right arm. Mike felt secure holding onto something while he stepped down a step. He found he could hold on to the end seat, walk down the step, get his balance, then grab hold of the next seat and so on. The process worked out nicely unless a person was sitting in the end seat and then Mike would grab hold of their arm, shoulder, or better yet, their head. We received some pretty strange looks on our quest to get to our seats. I apologized to many men who had their hat knocked off by sweet little Mike. The trek took us about thirty minutes. With a heat index of around 105, I was completely exhausted when we finally reached our seats. Mike and I sat down, wiped the sweat from our brows, and then he raised his chubby hands in the air and shouted "Yay, we did it!"

I had just begun to relax when Mike looked at me with his crooked lazy eye and said, "Mama, I go to bathroom a little bit?" Now anytime Mike mentioned that he needed to go to the bathroom we all knew that was an emergency signal to get him to the bathroom ASAP. When he stated that he needed to go a "little bit" that usually meant that he needed to go number one. Whenever he looked at you and said, "Uh oh, I go bathroom," that usually meant he had already gone number two and you were in big trouble. If he said, "My faucet's leaking," he had already gone number one. With Mike's new announcement, I immediately jumped out of my seat, took Mike by the hand, maneuvered him through our row, and turned to look up the incredibly long, immense concrete aisle we had just conquered. I looked up at the faces of people Mike had a short time ago held on to to get where we were and gulped, as I knew we were about to do it all over again, and then again when we headed back down the aisle to our seats. We somehow made it to the bathroom in time. I think focusing on the task before him made him forget for a few minutes that he had to go. We finally made it back down the massive concrete steps as I apologized once again and thanked the nice people for allowing Mike to use them as his support.

By now the game had started. We found our seats and settled in to enjoy the game. Just as we got comfortable a young man not far from us jumped the wall completely naked and began streaking across the outfield toward the infield. Every person in the stands stood up to see the entertainment. Mike stood and began to cheer. The naked man ran to second base and did a Pete Rose slide face first in the dirt. The entire crowd of forty thousand made the same "OHHHHHHH!" sound. The security guards were now chasing the man, who had gotten up and was running to right field. He reached the wall, jumped, and landed with his front side plastered to the wall. Again the entire crowd of forty thousand moaned, "OHHHHHHHHHH!" at the sight of a naked man smashed against the outfield wall. The security guards caught up to him, apprehended the streaker, handcuffed him, and walked him, in the nude, off the field.

My mom had tried desperately to cover the eyes of my children, who were trying anxiously to see the unforgettable image running on the baseball field. Brad and I were laughing at this unexpected sight. Mike, who did not realize that a naked man had just passed before him but thought something great had just happened due to the response of the crowd, raised his hands in the air and shouted, "Hallelujah, praise you Jesus, thank you good Lord!" People nearby looked at him rather strangely and sat down. I grabbed Mike by the belt loops and helped him down.

"This be fun, Mama."

I responded with, "It sure is, Mike; it's a full moon tonight." I looked up over the edge of the field to see a giant orange/red moon shining on us.

"It sure is," he said. "Two full moons tonight."

"That's right Mike, two full moons tonight," I laughed.

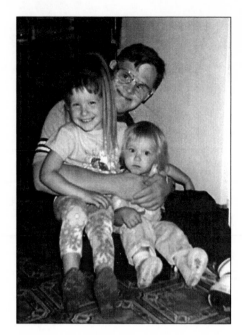

Mike with Whitney and Kaylee in 1992. They loved to sit on his lap.

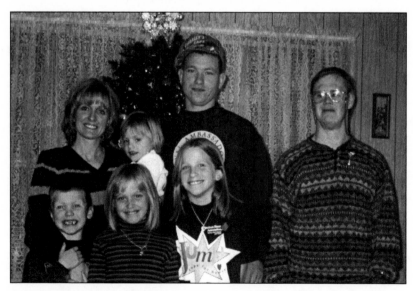

Christmas 1998 we were a big happy family.

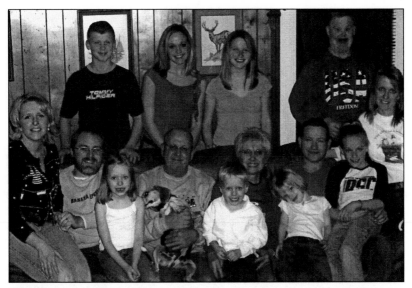

Christmas 2005 with my parents and sister's family. Mike loved being at Mom's house, especially during a holiday.

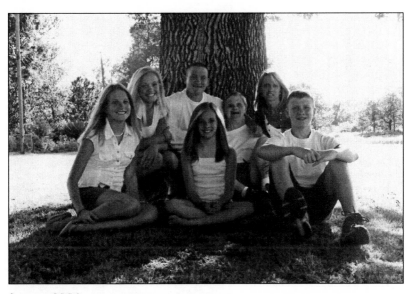

Summer 2006 in our backyard.

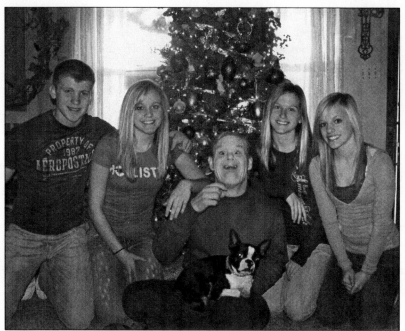

2007, our last Christmas with Mike.

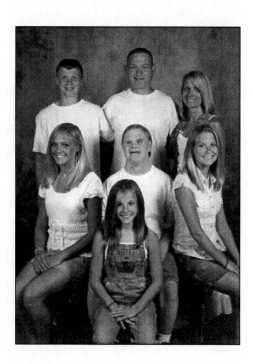

Mike was the center of our family.
We miss him terribly.

Chapter 22

Things Changed

We had been taking care of Mike for about nine or ten years when his behavior began to change. He started to repeat phrases over and over again. He would say, "My vacation's on already on," and "I'm getting married tomorrow." He would say them randomly all day long. He would take plastic bags and pack up his clothes and toiletry items and hide them around his room. He took food items like bananas and cookies from the kitchen and hid them in his bathroom medicine cabinet. He even started getting aggravated with me and would argue with me when I asked him to get ready for bed or shave his face.

After three or four months of Mike not acting like his kind, loving self, I took him to see a neurologist. The neurologist examined Mike and asked me some lengthy questions. The doctor then looked at me and simply said, "Mike is aging, and almost every Down's syndrome person gets Alzheimer's and dementia. As a matter of fact, every person with Down's syndrome who has had their brain autopsied had Alzheimer's lesions in their brain."

I sat in stunned silence. I looked at the doctor and asked with a choked, cracking voice how long Mike might have. "Maybe five years," was his response. I lowered my eyes and fought back the tears. "What now?" I asked. He referred us to his regular doctor for medication and explained that there was not much we could do to stop the aging process. I took Mike's hand and walked slowly out of the doctor's office. The forty-minute drive home was quiet and sad. I prayed for God to give us more than just five years with Mike. I also prayed that Mike would always know Brad, the kids, and me. I promised that as long as Mike was alive and I was able that I would take care of him.

We visited his regular doctor the next week and began a series of medications. Some worked and some did not. I began a search on the Web for information on adult Down's syndrome and was surprised by what I found. Most do not live to be as old as Mike, although many are living longer now because they are mainstreamed in society and well taken care of. They are no longer locked in facilities for the mentally ill. The doctor and I worked to keep Mike in tiptop shape. When he took the medicine he acted fairly normal. One thing I learned during my search on the Web was that people with Down's syndrome age twenty years faster than other people do. It was difficult to watch Mike age so quickly. He still loved everyone and had an incredible sense of humor, but no longer remembered things like family members' birthdays and anniversaries and all of the presidents' and first ladies' names.

I believe I was in denial as to how much he did age and how confused he was most of the time. I loved him as my own child and I never wanted him to go. I kept right on pushing him to keep up with us and to remember people and to pray. The doctor was wrong. We had Mike for eight years, not five. Those last three years are the most memorable. I think it was because we knew we did not have long with him, and we wanted to make every moment count.

Mike's hearty appetite remained the same; it just took him longer to eat. It also became increasingly difficult for him to make it to the bathroom. If you had asked me to clean up a grown person's messy underwear ten years ago, I would have instantly said, "NO!" I am amazed how God gave me the strength to clean Mike and care for him the way he needed and deserved. It is incredible how much I loved him. He would always look at me when I was cleaning him up and say, "I love you, Mama. You so beautiful."

When I went back to school to become a teacher my friends would tell me that I should go into nursing because "that is where the money was." I would respond by explaining that I did not like needles and I never wanted to clean up people's nasty poo. Well, as I have said before, God must have quite a sense of humor, because a few years later I was giving my youngest daughter and my husband seven shots a day due to diabetes and I was cleaning up Mike's poo. I know he did not mean to mess and wet his pants because the whole time I would be cleaning him up he would be saying "I so sorry, Mama; I love you." I would respond with, "I love you too, Mike, but please try to make it to the toilet, okay?"

"Okay, I sure will," was his reply.

As the months went by, it became worse. I prayed for him every time I had to be away for the night because Brad did not want to clean up a grown man's poo. God answered my prayers because no one ever had to clean up Mike's messes but me. I wanted to be the one to do it, and I did not want to inconvenience anyone. I realize now that every time I put on those rubber gloves and grabbed the bleach spray I was working for God. God had created Mike, and I was blessed to have him in my life. Cleaning him up was a part of worshipping my God. It was not easy. I became frustrated at times and wanted to cry many times when he messed right before we walked out the door for church or work. He was so precious though, and I know that if the roles had been reversed, Mike would have gladly cleaned up my messes.

A typical day for me went something like this: Get up at 5:20 to go run four miles, take a shower, get dressed, read my Bible, get Brad and the kids up for work and school, go into Mike's room, get him up, walk him to the toilet and hand him his cordless razor and tell him to shave "please." I would feed everyone breakfast, get Mike dressed, put his shoes on him, walk him into the kitchen, give him his medicine, walk him to the car, and then take him to my grandma's so I could go to work. I would teach third graders all day. I would pick the kids up from school and then go pick Mike up at 3:45, go home, and find some snacks for the kids and Mike. Help the kids with homework while I started cooking and then feed everyone supper. (This is if we did not have church, cheer practice, or a ballgame.) It was then time to bathe Mike and sit him on the toilet again. I would give him his medicine before bed, get the kids ready for bed, and then put Mike to bed. I made sure his nightlight was on, because he was afraid of ghosts, and told him good night. Every night for almost seventeen years he would tell me, after I told him good night, "I love you, Mama!" I love you too, Mikey Spikey," was my reply. Words cannot explain how much I miss hearing him say that. As crazy as my days went, ending them with Mike's loving words made it all worth it.

Chapter 23

The Flood

July 3, 2007, was another crazy day for the Douthit family. I woke up that morning and went for a run. As I passed some of my neighbors' houses, I noticed that the creek behind our homes, which was usually dry, especially during July in Oklahoma, was swelling with water and had crept into several backyards. I continued to run and noticed that two blocks away a few houses were starting to flood and people were moving out. I continued to run. My daily route was such that I went by the flooding houses twice before I headed home. When I came back around twenty minutes later the water had risen several feet. I reached home and looked into our backyard to check out the water. It was in the backyard, but that did not alarm me because it always got into the backyard after a heavy rain. By this time the kids were up and looking with me. They asked about the water and I assured them that we had nothing to worry about.

The phone began to ring. It was my neighbor in a panic. I assured her also that I had lived here for sixteen years and water had never been in the house so we would be fine. The phone rang again. It was my mother telling me that my grandparents' house was flooding and they needed help moving them. I gave the kids instructions. The older kids were to come with Brad and me to help move while Mackenzie and Mike were to stay at home. We headed out.

It was so sad to watch the panic, worry, and concern on my grandparents' faces as we were moving their precious things onto a trailer to be taken to our church for storage. In the middle of moving them my cell phone rang with my niece on the line stating that her house was about to flood. "Hold on," I told her. "We are on our way."

We found her standing on her porch holding her baby, watching the water rise up her steps. We began to move her things and to play with her son. I looked at my watch and remembered that I was to have exploratory surgery on my kidneys today and had to be at the hospital in ten minutes. I asked Kaylee to come with me so I could have someone drive me home after the procedure. We headed to the hospital, and I have to admit I was more than happy to be put to sleep on this crazy day.

I do not remember anything about the surgery except the doctor telling me that everything was fine with my kidneys. I do, however, remember recovery. Kaylee came in with my cell phone ringing. It was Mackenzie telling me that water was way up in the backyard. I once again assured her that we had nothing to worry about. She called back thirty minutes later informing me the water was now in the front yard and encircling the house. She sounded panicked. I looked at the nurse and explained that I needed to be unhooked from the IV because my house was about to flood. She tried her best to get me out of there, but it still seemed like an eternity, with the cell phone going off every few minutes informing me of the water conditions.

Kaylee and I finally drove up to our chaotic neighborhood. We could no longer park in front of the house due to the water. We found a place a half-block away and walked toward the house. I was shocked at the scene before us. In my watered down front yard were two large pickups with trailers hooked on the back and several exhausted people ready to help. I soon realized they were awaiting my okay to start moving things out. I was still very relaxed and loopy from the medicine the hospital had given me (thank the good Lord). I looked at everybody there, smiled, and said, "Sure, let's do it." Given the go-ahead, people went to work.

Remember, we had not moved in sixteen years. The last time we moved, we only had two children. It was crazy. I looked at Mike, who looked a little alarmed. He smiled at me and said, "Uh-oh, I go bathroom?" I took one look at him, sniffed the air, and realized we were too late to make it to the toilet. He needed a bath.

"Mike, why did you poop your pants?" I asked.

"Bob did it," he said.

"Bob did not poop in your pants, Mike," I replied.

"Yes, he did. B.O.B., he did it." I just laughed as I walked Mike slowly to his bathroom all the while dodging moving furniture and boxes. For some reason unknown to us he blamed everything on his cousin Bob. He did it so often that Whitney, Kaylee, and their boyfriends made T-shirts that simply said on the front, "Bob did it!"

I cleaned up Mike and put him in the bathtub. I did not think at the time that Mike understood what was really going on, that floodwaters were coming and we had to move. Several football players who were friends of the kids volunteered to help us. When they came into Mike's room to move his things, he stuck his head out of his tub and waved at them and smiled. "Hi good ol' buddies. I get married tomorrow."

"Hey Mike!" was their reply.

We finally had everything moved out. I looked around the house and fought back the tears. "God, please don't let our house flood. We just painted four rooms." With that said, Brad and I walked through the knee-high water to our van and headed to my parents' house where my grandparents and the kids awaited us. We lay down completely exhausted and fearful. Somehow we all drifted off to sleep.

We got up the next morning and headed back into town to check on our house. God blessed us greatly because the water only got into our garage and the sun porch. It did not get into the main part of the house. "Thank you, God, you are awesome," I kept repeating. Several of our neighbors were not so blessed. They had several inches of water in their homes. My grandparents had six inches in the lower part of their house, but it did not get into their upper living and sleeping area. My niece had wanted a new rental house anyway, so the timing was not bad for her. It took several months to restore the many houses that did flood. It was a tough year for many in our town.

The day after the flood, Mike started sitting and walking sideways. We tried several approaches to get him to sit and walk straight. I was afraid he had had a mini-stroke due to the stress of the flood. The doctor said he was fine and would be okay. He did straighten up a little, but continued to favor that same side. If he fell asleep in church, which he did often, he always leaned to the same side. I worried about him frequently and was very concerned. It seemed like he had aged several years overnight. I think all of us did that day, the day of the flood.

Two days later Mike and I had to go to the store. There was only one road in and out of our town due to the flood; therefore, the road was bumper to bumper and the cars were moving slowly. It was on this day that the alternator belt on my van decided to break. I was able to coast to a side road to get out of the endless traffic and pull under a shade tree. It was extremely hot. I looked in my rear view mirror to see Mike waving at me with his contagious smile. "I love you, Mama," he said.

"I love you too, Mikey Spikey. What are we going to do now?"

"We'll see time comes" was his famous response. I phoned our auto mechanic and explained our situation.

Within minutes the tow truck showed up; thank goodness he was on the other side of town. The mechanic chained my van up and looked at me and asked, "You two need a ride?" I looked at him and realized it would take Brad hours to get to us from our house in this slow traffic and the thought of us standing out in the heat was not appealing. I agreed to let him give us a ride; however, the tow truck was a semi. How would I ever get Mike up in the massive truck? "Mike," I said, "we are going for a ride, okay?"

"Okay, Mama," he said. I stood him next to the semi door and said, "Here we go, put your foot on the first step." He did and I grabbed his belt loop and hoisted him up. He sat in the middle of the truck right next to the driver. I climbed in and shut the door. I suddenly realized that I had never ridden in a semi and the look on Mike's face told me he hadn't either. Mike looked at the driver and said, "Hi, I Mike Douthit. I get married tomorrow."

"That's nice, Mike," the mechanic responded. He started that big rig and we headed out. Mike loved it. He waved and blew kisses to every car we passed. He really got excited when the mechanic blew the horn. Mike clapped and smiled. I am not sure what the mechanic thought of Mike and me, but I am pretty sure he will always remember us.

Chapter 24

The Fall

The older Mike got, the more trouble he had walking and he had many slow-motion falls. Falling wasn't hard on Mike, as he always fell very slowly; getting him up was the difficult part. On one occasion, Brad was taking Mike to the church to stay with Mom (she is the church secretary). They were walking up the handicap ramp with Brad leading the way. Suddenly Brad heard, "Daddy! Daddy! Help." Brad turned around to find Mike face down on the ramp with his head wedged between the concrete and the metal railing. To this day Brad still does not know how Mike got in that position. Brad scoped out the situation to determine the best way to rescue Mike. Brad tried pulling him out from the railing but his face was stuck. Brad went down the ramp to look at Mike's position from a different view. There lay Mike with his cute face smiling at Brad. Upon seeing Brad he instantly recited, "I love you, Daddy darling, you help me up!" "I'm trying, Mike," Brad replied. Brad decided to slowly lift back on Mike's head to remove his wedged face. When his face was released, Brad had to help Mike stand up; that was never easy. When Brad finally, slowly stood Mike up, he hugged Brad, laid his head on his shoulder, and said, "Thank you good ol' buddy! I love you, Daddy darling."

"I love you too, Mikey." Brad smiled and silently thanked God that Mike was not hurt.

On another occasion we were at a nearby lake with several teen-age friends of our children. Brad brought our boat and the kids were having a blast taking turns tubing behind the boat. Mike and I were sitting in lawn chairs on the shore watching. Mike was doing his famous cheering and blowing kisses to Brad and the kids while waving his undersized plump arms in the air shouting, "Go Daddy, go Sissy, go bubba Zeke, I love you, thank you Jesus!" Several other swimmers had walked by us, stared, and then realizing that Mike had Down's syndrome they would began to smile and chuckle and then wave at him.

Brad coasted the boat up to the shore to switch out the next rid-ers of the tube. Those of us watching walked up to the boat to hear the new "tubing story." Mike also stood up and began walking toward the boat. He yelled, "Hi Daddy, good ol' buddy," and we all turned to look just in time to see him, in complete slow motion, trip over a tree root that was sticking up through the rocks. Several of us tried to reach him before he fell forward, but watched in awe as he slowly rolled forward onto his oversized belly and rocked back and forth like the bottom of a rocking horse. We froze, awaiting a cry or a moan, but all we heard was, "Thank you, Jesus, I be okay." And, amazingly, he was fine, with only a small bruise on his knee. We helped him up and he smiled at us with his famous grin and stated, "I get married tomorrow!" At this we all exploded with laughter.

One day Mike and I were leaving Wal-Mart. I was ahead of him pushing the shopping cart while Mike was telling all the workers "bye" and that he was "getting married." Suddenly I heard, "Mama, help!" I turned around to find him lying on his face on the floor. I ran to him and discovered his shoestring had stuck in the grate in the front entrance of Wal-Mart. I removed the shoestring and began the difficult task of helping him up. He never could really help himself up so he was virtually dead weight when you lifted him. He may have been a small man, but he weighed around 200 pounds at this time (remember, he really liked to eat). I finally got him up, while several people walked past us and stared. He stood up on his feet, and we looked him over to check for bruises. He had none. He hugged me and said "Whoo, that hurt."

"I'm sure it did, Mikey," I responded. "Let's go home, Mike."

"Okay, I get married tomorrow?"

"Sure," I replied as we headed to the van.

Mike always seemed to bounce back from a fall without any injuries. I think that is why we were completely surprised on May 3, 2008. I had been mowing the yard on the rider. Kaylee had Mike outside in the backyard. She was on the trampoline while she and Mike played tag. She would run around in a circle on the trampoline while Mike stood on the ground and tried to tag her. "You it," he would laugh and call out. "You're it," Kaylee would reply. "No, you it," he would laugh. After several minutes of playing tag, she and Mike walked to the front yard and began racing. He was actually chasing her and jogging. We were all surprised to see him with so much energy. I laughed at them every time I drove the rider around to the front yard. It was a great, unforgettable afternoon with Mike.

I finally finished mowing the yard and drove the mower around the house. Kaylee had gone in the house, and Mike had wanted to stay in the yard to wait for me. I noticed Mike was sitting in the yard waving at cars that passed by. I told Mike to hang on and I would help him up after I put the mower away. I thought it strange for him to be sitting in the yard, but not a great deal surprised us about Mike. I walked toward him, took his hands, and began to pull. "OWWWWW!" he hollered.

"What's wrong?" I asked.

"It hurts."

"What hurts," I asked.

"I do not know," he responded.

"Why are you sitting in the yard, Mike?"

"I fell down," he replied.

"How did you fall down in the middle of the yard? There is nothing to trip over."

"I do not not not know," he added. I helped him up, but he would not put any weight on his right leg and held his right foot out to the side like it was asleep. I helped him into the house and set him on the couch. He fell asleep and I let him take a nap.

It was now bedtime and I told him to get up and get ready for bed. He could not get up. Brad was not home to help me. I tried to help him but he just sat down on the floor. I tried to get him up from the floor and he would holler in pain every time I tried to move him. When I asked him where it hurt, he would point to his foot, then to his back and then to his hip. I had no idea what was really wrong, as he could not give me a straight answer. I realized that I could not get him up and he was probably really hurt. I called 911 and waited for the ambulance. My kids stood around him with fear in their eyes. It was strange to see Mike like that. He was fine as long as you did not try to move him. He did not act like he was in constant pain and tried to grab the kids and give them a hug. I was afraid he had broken his hip. I remember wondering what we would do if he had a broken hip. How would we get him around and how would we take care of him?

The paramedics arrived and Mike welcomed them in with, "Hi, good ol' buddies." They checked him out and could not determine the cause of his pain. They decided to take him to the hospital in the ambulance. Every time they tried to move Mike he would say, "Be easy, okay, be easy." They honestly tried, but it still hurt him. He told all of them he was Mike Douthit and he was getting married to Becky tomorrow. They just smiled and told him that was nice. He was also strangely concerned about his shoe that we had removed. He kept asking the paramedics to take care of his shoe. They assured him his shoe would be fine. They had to lift him up, strap him in a chair, and carry him into the ambulance. I told them I would follow behind them in my van. I was planning on bringing Mike home as soon as we were finished in the ER. As I watched Mike being loaded into the ambulance for the trip to the hospital, I remember asking God, "God, is this the beginning of the end?" I also remember following very closely behind the ambulance so I could see what they were doing to him. I kept seeing them laugh and I knew that Mike was telling them funny stories

Mike had never before spent a night in the hospital. He was a very healthy guy considering his handicap. He had never broken a bone before this. That is why we are still not sure if his knee went out and he fell down, or if he fell down and hurt his knee. In any case, he had cracked his tibia, which is the bone right below the knee. I can't imagine what would have made him fall in the middle of the yard. I guess only God knows what really happened that afternoon. The doctor decided to secure his leg with a knee brace and admit him into the hospital until the bone specialist could see him. He was admitted around three o'clock in the morning. We settled into the room and tried to sleep. I was so worried about him that sleep was not an option. Mike, however, slept like a baby—a very loud, snoring baby, that is.

The nurses put in a catheter the next day so he would not have to get up to go to the bathroom. That is when the real trouble started. His kidneys started bleeding a lot. The kidney specialist was called in to see him, as was a medical doctor. They ran several tests and scans but could not determine what was causing the bleeding. He also had many, many bowel movements in his bed. Every time, I would put on the rubber gloves and help the nurses clean him up and bathe him. I learned some very helpful techniques for changing a person in bed, tips that helped me greatly when we brought him home.

We stayed in the hospital for seven days and seven nights. It was grueling for both of us. Mike had horrible apnea and snored loudly all day and all night. He hardly ever woke up during the day and hated it when the physical therapists tried to get him up and walk him. He pretty much refused, though he tried his best. They tied a belt around his waist and three physical therapists held him up to walk him. He did not want to walk so I would stand in front of him and promise him ice cream and cake if he would get up and take a few steps. He did okay the first few days, but he seemed to get weaker as the days went by.

My grandparents came to sit with him one day while I went to work. It was the last month of school and I had a lot of work to catch up on. The therapists came to walk Mike and he did not want to get up. My precious grandpa stood in front of him shouting, "Come on, Mike, you can do it." "Okay good ol' buddy. I try just a little bit, okay?" Mike responded, and he stood up and took a few steps for Grandpa Dareing.

I insisted on having someone there to feed Mike his meals when I had to be gone. He could no longer feed himself and I was convinced the nurses couldn't do it as well as I did. I only missed a few lunch meals, which Mom, Grandma, and Whitney gladly fed him for me. As I look back now, I am glad I was able to feed him because it made me sit down and really spend time with him three times a day during the last month of his life.

Spending seven days and seven nights in the hospital allowed me some much-needed time to reflect and think. I sat in a chair and stared at my Mike and reflected over the last seventeen years. I thought of how blessed we were for getting to share our lives with Mike. I began to thank God for all the years we had with him and for how many laughs we had, and for how Mike had made us see the world differently through new eyes. Because of his love for everyone, we learned the importance of love and life through a mentally retarded man. I chuckled inside as I realized I no longer saw Mike as being retarded. He was my son and I loved him just like I loved and cared for my other four children. I prayed we would have Mike for many more years. Deep inside I knew my prayers would not be answered the way I wanted them to be.

Mike's kidneys finally stopped bleeding and we were finally allowed to take Mike home, in a wheelchair, with Depends, and to a hospital bed. It was not easy to accept.

Our pastor helped me take Mike to the doctor a few days later to get a cast put on his leg. They had left his knee brace on until the swelling went down. Pastor Jinks lifted Mike from the chair to the van, then back into the chair to go to the doctor's office. Each time he lifted him up Mike would put his arms around him and try to kiss him on the neck. Our pastor would just laugh at him and say, "Mike, you're not supposed to kiss men." Mike would smile and say, "I love you, good ol' buddy."

Mike once again charmed the receptionist and the nurses with his smile and kind charm. His knee was still swollen and the doctor removed several vials of fluid off his knee. He told the doctor he wanted a blue cast because it would match his blue eyes. The doctor agreed and put a blue cast on Mike's leg. They gave him a walking cast in hopes that Mike would walk on his own. (It did not work.)

Our pastor helped me bring him home where we all signed his cast and drew smiley faces on it. He thought it was pretty neat. He looked really cute with his blue cast, sitting in his hospital bed with a huge grin on his adorable face.

Chapter 25

May

The month of May was a crazy blur. Our lives changed drastically as we struggled and adjusted to caring for Mike. He tried so hard to act normal and keep up with us, but we slowly realized that he was not behaving the same. He still had his wit about him, but his strength was gone. Whitney was finished with her semester of college, which was wonderful because I had three more weeks of teaching, and I needed her to stay with Mike until summer vacation. Whitney was a trooper. She did a wonderful job of taking care of Mike. She fed him lunch and helped the nurse's aide and the physical therapist lift him and bathe him. I am so very proud of her. She proved her adulthood that month.

A physical therapist came by twice a week, but soon gave up because Mike would not stand up for him and absolutely refused to walk. When I stood him up he would walk for me to his chair and even to the toilet. I guess Mike just did not trust the therapist. A nurse's aide also came to help bathe Mike three times a week. Whitney and I made sure one of us was always there to help her because Mike would not walk for her. He was so sweet to her, though. He always had a smile for her and a hug. She fell instantly in love with him, like everyone seemed to. She put lotion on him and made him look quite handsome.

I would get him up in the mornings and walk him to the toilet. It was a difficult and exhausting task for both of us, but I had so much hope that if I got him out of bed and walked him three times a day he would eventually get better. I would sit him on the toilet and hand him his razor while I picked out clean clothes for him and prepared his breakfast. I did not have much time in the mornings because I was still teaching school. I would then put clean clothes on him, including his Depends, which was hard to accept because Mike had always been so good with toileting in his earlier years. I would then have Zeke feed Mike his breakfast while I finished getting ready for work. Mike adored Zeke and enjoyed having Zeke feed him. Zeke also cherished Mike. Not many fifteen-year-olds can say they fed a fifty-five-year-old man who was sitting on the toilet breakfast every morning before school. Zeke never once complained.

We would then walk him back to his bed, sit him up, and turn the TV to the oldies station. Mike loved *The Beverly Hillbillies, Andy Griffith, The Three Stooges,* and *Happy Days.* Our little Boston terrier puppy would climb up on Mike's bed and lay beside him while he rubbed her back. She loved him and he adored her. I would kiss him on the forehead and tell him good-bye. He would ALWAYS say, "Bye, Mama, I love you." "I love you too, Mikey Spikey," was my morning reply, and I headed off to work with Mike in Whitney's care and concern on my mind.

May 10, 2008 started out as a normal Saturday with Mike. I got him dressed and began the menial task of getting him into our kitchen. We had built him a very nice large bedroom and a new dining room off of our kitchen. In order to build the add-on we could only leave a 25-inch doorway due to the structure of the kitchen window. Walking through the doorway was never a problem, but getting a wheel chair through the door was next to impossible. To get Mike to his bedroom and back through the kitchen, we had to stand him up, collapse the wheel chair, roll it through the doorway, walk him through, and then sit him back in the chair. It was difficult enough with two people, doing it by yourself was close to unfeasible. So, on this beautiful day in May, Brad and I got Mike to the kitchen table for breakfast. He played with the kids and then ate lunch. We then put him back in his bed for a nap. My sister in law had scheduled a family dinner for that evening. Brad and the kids went and I decided it would be too much for Mike so he and I stayed home. Sometime during the afternoon the weather began to change. Black clouds rolled in, the wind changed directions, and the temperature dropped very rapidly. In Oklahoma when the wind changes directions and the temperature drops, everyone goes outside to look for a tornado funnel. I was no exception. While Mike snored away I went out the door to take a look. It was at this moment that the tornado sirens began to blow. I went back in the house and wondered what I should do with Mike. We needed to get in the center of the house away from windows. I woke him up, put him in the chair, wheeled him to the kitchen doorway, and began the task of getting him through the 25-inch outlet. I stood him up and as I tried to collapse the wheel chair we began to fall. We both slowly slid down onto the kitchen floor with tornado sirens blasting in the background. I sat him up and tried to get him in his chair to no avail. I sat beside him, looked into his precious blue eyes and said, "Mike a tornado is coming, if you go, I go." He smiled at me and replied, "We go together, okay Mama." Then he bowed his head and prayed.

The tornado passed over us and headed to a small local town known as Picher, Oklahoma where it caused devastating damage. Several lives were lost and hundreds of homes were destroyed. I know God spared us that day as Mike and I sat in our kitchen floor praying.

We were able to take Mike to church a few times after his accident. It was quite a chore to get him in the car, taking at least two people. It also wore him out and I did not want to push him too hard. I could tell by the looks on the church members' faces when they saw Mike that they were concerned. It was as if he had aged twenty years in a just a few weeks. He let us push his wheelchair around and never once tried to get up.

The first Sunday we took him to church, Brad was pushing his chair down the aisle. He spotted Grandma and grabbed hold of the pew she was sitting in and would not let go. He wanted to sit beside her as he did every Sunday, but we wanted him to sit with us so we could keep a close eye on him. Brad explained to him that he would be sitting by us. He sighed very loudly and said, "Help us, Good Lord!" We laughed at him and pushed him down the aisle. He continued to lean to the left very badly and it was hard to keep him sitting in his chair, as he would also fall asleep easily.

The last Sunday we took him to church started out like a usual crazy Sunday for us. I walked Mike to the toilet but noticed that he never wanted to use his good leg anymore and never wanted to put any weight on his hurt leg. I was dressing him when suddenly he acted like he was having a seizure. He rolled his head back and forth and slumped forward. I held his head back and talked to him. At first he could not respond, but soon he looked at me and smiled. I know it only lasted a few seconds, but it scared me very badly. He snapped out of it just as quickly as it had begun. I talked to him and he seemed to be fine. I wondered if his medicine had had an effect on him.

He acted fairly normal the rest of the day, just a little tired. We went to Mom's to eat dinner, and he ate fine. He looked at Mom and said, "You such a good cook. Like mother like daughter." I am sure he was referring to Grandma and Mom, not Mom and me.

Chapter 26

Hard Days

We took him home after dinner and put him in his hospital bed to rest. I was very concerned about him because I was to leave that afternoon to drive five hours away to southern Oklahoma for a teacher-training seminar for National Boards. I would not be back until Tuesday evening. I gave very strict instructions to the family, made a list of responsibilities they each had in caring for Mike, and put Mike's medicine in a medicine holder for each day. I got in the car and headed off wondering what the future held for my family.

I can't explain the strange burden I had in my chest as I drove across the state of Oklahoma. Dad insisted I take Mom's new small car because it got thirty-five miles to the gallon. With gas prices rising daily, I gladly agreed. I prayed all the way to my destination and I felt God talking to me. He clearly told me that we would lose Mike this summer. I, of course, tried to argue with God, but I knew He was preparing me for a huge loss. I tearfully pleaded with God and sent up two prayer requests.

1. I asked God to please allow me to be there when Mike went to heaven.

2. I asked God to please not let Mike lay in a bed being a vegetable for months and months.

The thought of putting him in a nursing home and letting other

89

people take care of him terrified me. Realistically, however, how long could I take care of him if he ever did become bedridden? What would I do with him when school started in August? Many questions loomed in my head and my heart. I suddenly understood the verse in the book of Luke, chapter 2 verse 19, that says, "And Mary kept all of these things and pondered them in her heart."

I needed a break from wondering. I reached in the CD holder and grabbed one of Mom's CDs and popped it in the stereo. It just happened to be Martina McBride, one of my favorites. I was singing along with her, having a good time and trying not to think about losing Mike when my favorite song came on, "God's Will." The girls and I love this song because it reminds us so much of Mike. It tells of a handicapped boy named Will who changed a family's life. The first line and the last line of the song say, "I met God's Will on a Halloween Night, he was dressed as a bag of leaves." I sang the entire song with Martina until it came to the last line. For the first time, as I listened to her say, "I met God's Will on a Halloween night," I abruptly burst into tears. I suddenly recalled that Mike had moved in with us on a Halloween night. He was my little spook.

I cried all the way along the highway through Oklahoma City. When I finally gathered myself together, I told God and myself that "God's Will" must be played at Mike's funeral. I gasped as I realized that I had just said, "Mike's funeral." What a horrendous thought. How could I even think about it? What would we ever do without him? Surely this was not going to happen soon. I thanked God for talking to me and told Him that I believed He would grant my two requests to be right beside Mike when he went to heaven and not to allow Mike to become bedridden.

I made it to Ardmore, Oklahoma, and was able to stay with my Aunt Terri and Uncle Robert, who ended up being a strong support for me for the next few days. When I arrived, I called home to check on Mike and the kids. They said Mike was doing fine and had enjoyed his supper. I explained to Whitney that I had made arrangements for the nurse to come around 8:30 in the morning to help her get Mike up, clean him, and get him in his wheelchair. The nurse usually did not come until around 11:00, but she agreed to come early since I had to be gone.

That night I spent most of the night awake praying for Mike and my family. I could not sleep and thought I was just nervous about my seminar. When I can't sleep I always assume God is urging me to pray. I awoke around 5:00 A.M., confused and anxious. My aunt sat down with me to eat breakfast and agreed to pray for me and promised to have a wonderful supper when I came back that evening.

I signed in at my seminar around 8:30 and had just sat down in the large conference room when my cell phone began to vibrate. I looked at the number and saw that it was from home. I hesitated to answer it, figuring it was Mackenzie telling me Zeke had drunk the last of the milk. Then I remembered that Brad, Zeke, and Mackenzie had gone early to my in-laws where they were planning to spend the week camping for Brad's vacation. I decided to answer the call.

I walked out of the conference room into the commons area and said, "Hello."

"MOM, Mike is not doing so good. He is acting weird and breathing hard. The nurse and I got him up and sat him on the portable toilet and he just started acting strange," Whitney's panicked voice sounded in the phone.

"Let me talk to him," I directed. I could tell by the sound of Mike's breathing he was having a panic attack. "Mike, this is Mama, calm down and breathe slowly," I pleaded. "Okay, Mama," was his response, and for a few seconds he calmed down. The nurse got on the phone and stated that he did not look good and they were trying to get him back in the bed. I told them to call me back when they got him calmed down.

I went back into the conference, sat down, and the phone vibrated again. It was the nurse stating that Mike's blood pressure was a little low and asking me what we should do. I told her to check it again and if it was higher then I could get my friend who was a nurse to come over and watch him. She said that she would and we hung up. I went back to the conference only to get back up to answer my phone. It was Kaylee's good friend Matt informing me that things were not looking good and I could hear Whitney and Kaylee crying in the background. Matt explained that Mike had had a seizure and stopped breathing. The nurse was trying CPR and the paramedics were on the way. I hung up and froze. The world around me began to spin and spin and spin.

Time stood still as I pictured in my mind what was going on at my home while I was five hours away. I went to the main coordinator of the Oklahoma State National Boards and told her my situation. She felt sorry for me but explained that if I left I would lose my $2500 scholarship and could not work on my National Boards. I had been denied the scholarship the previous year and knew this was a huge honor. I stared at her and walked outside. I called home. "What is going on?" I asked in a panic. Brad and Zeke had made it to the house and Brad explained that the paramedics were working on Mike and it did not look good. I called back in five minutes. Brad answered and explained that they were taking Mike out of the house to the ambulance. I will never forget his words as he said, "He's gone. I think we lost him."

I stood dumbfounded. I was shaking all over my entire body. I just stood there immobile for what seemed like forever. I finally looked to heaven and said, "God, I asked you to let me be there when he died. I wanted to be holding his hand when Jesus came and got him. How could this happen with me being so far away? This just doesn't make sense. My family needs me. What should I do?" I called my Uncle Robert and he told me to take some deep breaths and try to stay calm and not to leave just yet. At that moment my phone rang on the other line. It was my dad. I slowly answered, afraid of what he had to say. "We have a heartbeat," he stated excitedly. "We have a heartbeat." He told me that Mike was not responsive, but had a strong heartbeat. He also told me not to come home unless something else happened. Then my dad ended with, "We are just playing the waiting game right now. Mike won't go until his mama gets here." I burst into tears. Mike had a heartbeat. They had lost him for forty-four minutes but now he had a strong heartbeat. I once again looked toward heaven and thanked God for keeping Mike alive. "Please God, help him hold on until I get there," I pleaded.

I still do not know how I made it through that two-day seminar. Well, I do know I had my entire family and church praying for me. I had very little focus and probably did not get much out of the conference, but I kept my scholarship. The doctor was to come on Monday night to inform us of Mike's condition. I asked my sister to put me on speakerphone so I could be a part of the discussion. The doctor walked in, looked at the large number of people in the waiting room, and marveled that everyone was there for Mike. There were at least twenty family members and friends there for Mikey. He explained that Mike had two blood clots. One in each lung, and one was very large. They could send him to a bigger hospital and do surgery, but he would probably not survive the trip, or they could give him some high-powered medicine to try and dissolve the clots. However, he had been with very little oxygen for forty-four minutes, and they were not sure of the extent of brain damage he might have. They also did not know how Mike's body would handle things because they had never dealt with a person with Down's syndrome who was as old as Mike. The doctor did not know what would happen, but he assured us that Mike's heartbeat was still strong.

I felt a little better after hearing from the doctor. Brad assured me he and Zeke would stay the night with Mike and would keep a close eye on him and would inform me of any changes. I went to bed and once again spent the entire night tossing and praying. It was during this time I felt God pick me up and hold me in his arms. I knew he was carrying me and would not put me down until He knew I was ready.

I made it through the next grueling day. I decided to fast and pray until I could see Mike again. The conference ended at 4:00, and I was pulling out of the parking lot at 4:03. I had just reached the interstate highway heading north when I received a text message. It was from my good friend Ruth. It simply said, "May angels protect you and bring you home safely." I smiled as I thought about the loss of her mother only three months earlier on Easter morning. She understood how I felt and knew I needed prayer at that exact moment.

The ride home was grueling. I was not tired, but I was wired. I kept calling my family asking how Mike was doing and they assured me he was waiting for me and everything would be fine. I prayed the entire trip, thanking God that Mike was still alive. I made it home in four hours and thirty minutes. I was so relieved to see the Miami exit. I had made it. God had carried me home.

I quickly entered the hospital and practically ran to ICU. My family greeted me with hugs and ushered me into Mike's room. It is difficult to put into words how I felt when I saw Mike. He was attached to numerous tubes and machines. He looked swollen and he was constantly drooling and oozing bubbles out of his mouth where the breathing tubes were. He was hooked up to a breathing machine, life support really, but was breathing some on his own. I walked over to him, took hold of his hand, put my head on his chest, looked up into his closed eyes, and whispered, "It's okay, Mike, Mama is here and I love you." I stayed in that position for quite a while thanking God for my years with Mike.

The ICU nurses were wonderful. They were quiet and gentle and seemed to understand our thoughts and feelings. They even pulled in a recliner right next to Mike's bed so I could spend the night with him. How often does that happen in ICU? I encouraged my exhausted family to go home and get some rest. My sister volunteered to stay the night in the waiting room in case I needed her. She really *knew* I needed her. She is truly a saint and I am very, very thankful for her.

I spent the night holding Mike's hand and wiping the bubbly slobbers coming out of his mouth. I slept very little, but felt rested. It was so good to touch Mike's warm hand and know his heart was still beating, but questions lingered in my mind: Will Mike make it? How long does he have? Will he recover and be like he used to be? Will I be able to care for him? What will we do without him? I couldn't take it anymore. I looked at the clock and saw that it was 5:25 A.M. I needed some air. I walked to the waiting room and woke my sister. She said she would sit with Mike, and outside I went.

I began to jog and pray. The sun was beginning to come up and was shining some light through the clouds. I looked to the western sky and the clouds had formed a beautiful sculpture that looked just like angel wings. I stared at the incredible sight before me and asked aloud, "Oh, Jesus, are you sending your angels to get Mike today?" The song "Surely the Presence of the Lord is in this Place" started playing in my head. I sang it the entire way. I finished my jog and headed back to the hospital refreshed, encouraged, and terrified.

I entered Mike's room and found my sister leaning over his bed reading the Bible to him. He still had not responded to us, but I believe he heard every word we said. She offered to go downstairs and get us some breakfast. After she left I also noticed that Mike was no longer drooling like he had been. I asked the nurse about it and she looked at me and simply said, "Angie, I don't know. I have never in the twelve years I have been working in ICU had a person this old with Down's syndrome. I really don't know what to tell you."

She left, and I sat in a chair next to Mike. I took his swollen hand in mine, leaned down to his face, and whispered to him, "Mike, it is okay to go to heaven. We will be just fine and I know we will see you soon. When you get there please tell my grandma Trask and my uncle Danny hello and please thank your mother for raising such a wonderful person and for allowing me to be your mama for seventeen years." Wait a minute. My thoughts began to race. What was the date? I looked at my watch. It was June 4. Oh no! My uncle Danny, who was the rock of our family and who had spent twenty-three years in a wheelchair due to complications from his service in Vietnam, died six years ago on June 4. How will my grandma handle losing Mike on the same day that she lost her son? It was also my sister's oldest daughter's birthday today. I looked to heaven and said, "God, you are in control of everything and I know you have this day under control. Please take care of my precious grandma and help her through today."

I looked up to see my mom walking around the corner and my sister returning with breakfast. The nurse walked in and said that the doctor should be in pretty soon. I called Brad and Zeke but they were already on their way. Mike had some cousins who had been visiting and were greatly concerned about his well-being. They were also on their way. The doctor came in, looked Mike over, studied the readings on his machines, sighed, looked down, then looked into my eyes and said, "It won't be long." I sat in a chair beside Mike, held his hand, put my head on his arm and stared at him.

The doctor explained that we needed to make some decisions about releasing him from the machines. Although his heart seemed strong, he was still not breathing on his own and his pupils were not responding to light. He told us to think about it and he would be back shortly to discuss options with us. Mom began calling family members telling them they had better come to the hospital if they wanted to tell Mike good-bye.

Mom phoned Grandma and Grandpa. Grandpa answered, listened to mom, and told her that Grandma just couldn't handle it today. She was having a hard time. We all understood. Mom told him to take care of Grandma and to give her the message and to please pray.

Mike's cousin showed up and we began to explain to her what the doctor had told us. She did not believe us and wanted to talk to the doctor. The nurse called him and the doctor came to Mike's room. I was still holding Mike's hand with my head on his arm, tears rolling down my face uncontrollably. The doctor explained that Mike did not have long and that he should not be kept alive on machines. He looked at us and said, "I have an older uncle with Down's syndrome. I would never want him kept alive this way. It's not fair to him." Mike's cousin was not ready to make a decision. I silently prayed that we would not have to make any decisions, that God would come and get Mike without him having to suffer any longer. I opened my eyes and noticed that my mom and sister were also praying. I learned later they were praying the same prayer.

By now Whitney and Kaylee had made it, and Kaylee's friend had left to get Mackenzie from her friend's house. We all gathered around Mike's bed and cried. I always knew this moment would come someday, but none of us were ready for it. He was the joy in our home. The one who made all of us laugh at times when we did not feel like laughing. He was the one that always told us he loved us. The one who told me I was beautiful. The one who thought I was a good cook. The one who applauded everything we did. The one who said, "Woooo-weeeee, you look so nice!" when we were dressed up for a special event. The one who truly understood who God was. The one who never met a stranger. The one who hugged everybody. The one who understood the importance of family and friends. The one who was loved by every dog we ever met. The one who brightened up any room. What would we ever do without Mike? I looked up and couldn't believe my eyes when I saw my grandma and grandpa enter the room. Grandma walked right up to Mike's bed and smiled. She couldn't stay away. The woman is a rock. Her strength amazes me.

The doctor had been watching Mike's machines carefully and said simply, "The machines just took over on his breathing." Where he had been breathing on his own, he was now breathing solely on a machine. My mom and grandma began singing aloud "When We All Get to Heaven." As they sang I noticed a tear begin to roll down Mike's left cheek. I will never forget the words they sang: "When we all get to heaven, what a day of rejoicing that will be, when we all see Jesus, we'll sing and shout the victory!" My mom looked at Mike with tears in her eyes and said, "Shout the Victory, Mike!" A tear rolled down his other cheek. His heart stopped beating, and he was gone. He was gone!

The nurse came and began turning off the machines and just like that Mike was in heaven. None of us had to make any decisions to turn off the machines. God just sent his angels to come and get him.

I continued to hold his hand as one by one every family member and friend came to his bedside and kissed him good-bye, tears streaming down their faces. I stayed until everyone was in the hall-way. I laid my body across his and hugged him. He was still warm and it was hard to believe he was gone. I stayed there crying, telling him good-bye and how much I loved him and would miss him until my grandpa came and took me by the shoulders and walked me out of the room. I couldn't stop crying. I usually do not cry, but this was out of my control. I walked to the waiting room where my family and friends were, and then the elevator opened and out walked Mackenzie and Matt. I grabbed her and told her Mike was gone. She began sobbing, saying "No, he can't be, he just can't be gone." I held her and cried some more.

We gathered in the waiting room awaiting our next move. I noticed Whitney and Kaylee sitting on the waiting room couch, crying. I squeezed in between them, put my thin arms around each of them, and held them while we cried some more. I looked across the room at Zeke. He had his head in his hands. My heart broke for him. I remembered the day we brought Zeke home from the hospital and how proud Mike was of his new brother. Now Zeke had just lost his only brother.

I looked around the room at all the teary-eyed faces and wondered how we would ever get through this. Then I remembered the requests I had made to God: 1. That I could be there when Mike went to heaven; and 2. That he would not lie in a bed for months not knowing who we were. I looked to heaven and thanked God for his goodness and loving kindness. I then looked at my grandma and tried to imagine her pain on this June 4 and wondered why out of 365 days in the year Mike was to die on the same day as my Uncle Danny had died. I came to the conclusion that God must have set aside this special day to bring incredible men to heaven. I missed Mike already.

Mike's family began planning the funeral and asked me about pallbearers. I gave them my list and they gladly obliged. The hospital chaplain came out and told us we could visit Mike again. I asked if they could cut his cast off. For some reason, I wanted to keep it. Mothers covet strange things like that. They said they would if we would wait a few minutes. We did and then they let us walk in to see him.

It was amazing. The tubes were gone. He looked twenty years younger. All of his wrinkles were gone. His hands and face were filled out and he looked to be at total peace. Wow! What a difference. It is amazing how seeing Jesus can completely change the look on your face.

We told him good-bye again and then left so the funeral home could take him. Mike's family made preparations for us to meet at the funeral home to make arrangements for his funeral. They asked me to bring one of his favorite suits, a tie, and a picture for the paper. I gathered my things and realized that I was leaving the hospital without him, without my Mikey Spikey. Whoa. ... That was a hurtful slap in the face.

Chapter 27

Going Home

I walked in our quiet house and went straight to Mike's room. We had let the dog in and she had run immediately to his bed, climbed up, and laid down waiting for Mike to lie down and rub her back. I could not take seeing her lie there waiting for Mike. I fought back the tears. I grabbed the phone, called the facility that had brought the bed and wheelchair and asked them to please come and get them as soon as possible. They were there in thirty minutes. I helped them carry the items out, crying the entire time.

I picked out a nice suit and my favorite tie and let the girls choose a picture of Mike for the paper. I showered and dressed for the funeral home. I felt like a robot. I was moving but not thinking. It was bizarre.

I left the kids with the task of collecting every picture we had of Mike to prepare a PowerPoint show of his life for the funeral. Mike had all of his baby and childhood pictures in his room, upon the backs of which he had proudly written "Michael Bradley Dale Douthit." I thought a slide show of Mike's life would be nice for the funeral and felt it would be good for the kids to go through Mike's pictures.

Brad and I managed to arrive at the funeral home on time carrying Mike's suit and tie. I sat down in a chair around a table to discuss funeral arrangements with his family. I had never done this before. I had never realized how many decisions there were. Our pastor showed up to offer his support and we were happy to see him. Mike's family was wonderful about allowing me to select the location of the funeral, the songs, and the order of the funeral. We decided to ask Mike's pastor from First Assembly of God church to give the eulogy and our pastor would speak. I also felt led to share our story of how we got Mike and how much he meant to us. I had never spoken at a funeral. Was I crazy? How could I get through it? It didn't matter. I would do anything for Mike. I felt he deserved one last statement of the wonderful life he gave us. Then I remembered the song "God's Will." It had to be played at his funeral. I wanted everyone to see how precious Mike was to us and how weird it was that we got him on Halloween night like the song stated.

We picked out a beautiful blue casket that I knew he would love because it was his favorite color—"Just like my eyes," he would say. Embroidered inside the lid were the words "Going Home." We all agreed it was perfect for him and did not realize until we were at the graveside that the headstone his mother had selected Mike and herself almost twenty years earlier had the words "Going Home" engraved on it. It was affirmation that once again God was guiding us through this whole process.

Brad and I drove home in silence. We walked into a home already full of plants and food. Our family, church family, and neighbors had heard of our loss and were offering their condolences. We were very grateful. The kids were excited to be getting anything other than my famous frozen food. People poured in and out offering hugs and smiles. It was comforting to know so many people cared about our extreme loss. Whitney had collected the pictures she found of Mike and headed to our preacher's house to begin the tedious process of scanning them into the computer for the Power-Point. We looked at the pictures before she left and laughed at the fun memories of Mike. It was good not to be crying. I realized we would somehow get through this.

Chapter 28

The Funeral

We were allowed to view Mike's body the next day. Brad, the kids, my mom, and I stood there in amazement at how wonderful Mike looked. He looked happy. He looked much younger and reminded us of how he had looked when we first started caring for him. We were all impressed and told the funeral home how incredible he looked. The navy blue suit matched perfectly the blue of his casket and his pretty eyes.

We placed a flashlight in the casket for him because he asked his family after his mother's funeral if he could have a flashlight and an air conditioner with him when he died. I could not fit an air conditioner in the casket, but we found a nice flashlight. My mom had purchased a boutonnière for him to be placed on his lapel. She wanted him to look like he was going to the wedding he never got to have. He looked precious and perfect.

The next evening was the visitation night for friends and family. It was wonderful. Everyone looked at Mike's body and stated how young he looked and how all of his wrinkles were gone. I received many encouraging hugs and condolences. I replied that I would miss him greatly, but that I was so happy for him. He was in heaven with Jesus, and he would not come back here if I asked him to. We were overwhelmed with the heartening response of so many people.

We headed home to prepare ourselves for the funeral. I felt numb. I've been to many funerals and wondered how the families had gotten through them. I understood now they were just moving on the outside, but hurting beyond belief on the inside.

The funeral took place at our church the next day. I felt it was fitting since Mike had grown up going to church in the same building and had been baptized there. The women of the church fed us a delicious meal that Mike would have loved. We then walked into the sanctuary for the funeral.

The church was filled with friends and family. I let Mike's biological family sit in the first pew and my family sat in the next one. When the last person sat down, the PowerPoint began. We had 130 pictures, which allowed for two songs to be played along with the slide show. We started with "I Can Only Imagine" and ended with "Another Time and Another Place" by Sandi Patty and Wayne Watson. It was astonishing. Whitney had done a perfect job of displaying Mike's entire life from beginning to end. People in the audience laughed and cried at the adorable pictures of Mike. The last picture showed Mike with a sailor's hat on, saluting. It was as if he was saying good-bye to us all. The girls had also put together a page of "Mike quotes" that were handed out as people entered. They were cute and refreshing.

Brother Baser stepped to the podium and shared several wonderful stories of Mike's life as a young man, many of which I had never heard. It was so nice to listen to the funny things Mike did when he was younger. Brad squeezed my shoulder as we both wished we had known Mike when he was a child and teenager. Brother Baser finished and we played a recorded version of my mom singing "Hallelujah Square." It was then my turn.

As I walked up the steps to the podium, I prayed that God would speak through me. I looked at the familiar faces in the crowd, took a deep breath, and began. I told them how we had gotten Mike on Halloween Night and what a blessing he had been to our lives. I told them that I had told Brad that he would have to pick up the slack now because I was used to being told, "I love you. You so beautiful," by Mike every day and I was not ready for it to end. I told of how Mike helped me with our children and day care kids when they were little and how our kids had helped me take care of him the last few years. I told them how Mike never forgot a birthday or an anniversary and how he loved having birthday parties and blowing out his candles. I told them how much Mike loved Jesus and what a great job his mother did raising him in church and how he would look at people being rude or cussing and say aloud, "They need Jesus, Mama." I also explained the story of Camden's mom at Wal-Mart and how Mike had impacted her. I told of how Mike inspired everyone he met and how thankful we were to have had the privilege of caring for Mike. I then read an essay Mackenzie had written in fifth grade. It went like this:

I have a hero. It is my brother Mike Douthit. My mom and dad got him when he was in his late 30's. His parents both died. He was old enough to take care of himself but he has Down's syndrome so he can't really take care of himself. I've known him since I was born.

He is my hero, one because I never thought I would see such an amazing guy as him. He really is amazing. Down's syndrome people are not supposed to live as old as fifty-three. That is how old Mike is this day and he is still up and going, as in walking, talking, laughing, singing, and all sorts of things. He's a miracle.

Another thing about Mike is that he can make you feel happier than any other thing in the world. An example is, one day I got in big trouble for back mouthing my mom and dad so I got a spanking and got sent to my room for two hours. I never thought I would be happy again. I tried every thing to cheer myself up. I even tried listening to music. It didn't help at all. Not one bit. I kept on listening to it though. Then the door opened and there was Mike, my hero, just dancing to that music like he had never danced before. It made me feel very happy.

It made me feel a lot happier than before. And, that is another reason he is my hero.

Another reason Mike is my hero is because I'm one of those person's who loves to laugh. And if you live with Mike, you can laugh all day long. Practically every sentence he says makes you want to burst out laughing. That is another reason Mike is my hero.

In my book Mike is not Down's syndrome. He's a normal person just like everybody else, except he's my HERO!

I finished by telling them that I thank God for every single day my family was allowed to share with Mike. I also told them that I know it was God's will for us to take care of Mike, our little spook who we got on Halloween Night.

The song "God's Will" by Martina McBride followed. I heard several joyful sniffles as people cried happy tears. It was very bittersweet. We knew we would all miss Mike, but were so happy for him. He was in heaven with Jesus. It just doesn't get any better than that.

Our pastor then spoke and shared how much Mike meant to the church and to his own family. He concluded by stating how much Mike loved Jesus and how he had wanted everyone to know Him. We ended the service with our friend Jolene singing "Surely the Presence of the Lord Is in This Place." It was a beautiful service. Mike would have loved having all of this attention. He would have been very pleased with everything.

Everyone came by and hugged us and told us how sorry they were and how blessed Mike had been to have a family's love like we gave him. I would reply by saying that we were the ones who were blessed. As I was hugging everyone, two tiny arms grabbed me around the waist and I heard the precious words, "I love you, Mrs. Douthit." It was one of my third-grade students. He had heard all the "Mike stories" I had told in class and knew I would be sad that he was gone. What a blessing to have him and his mother there.

Next, Brad, the kids, and I had to ride in the funeral's family car. It was the first time for all of us. We sat close and quiet. It would be hard to put Mikey in the ground, but I reminded all of us that it was only his body. He was really in heaven.

We gathered around his grave and sang "I'll Fly Away." I pictured him singing it with us in heaven using his "sign language."

Chapter 29

Life without Mike

We came home to a quiet house. Our family and friends had to go home. It was over. Mike's funeral was over. He was gone. I walked to his room, sat in his favorite chair, rocked back and forth, closed my eyes and fought back the tears.

I had always thought after the funeral was over things got better and life went on. Well, I was wrong. Every day seemed to get worse. I found myself going to the kitchen to get his medicine at bedtime, only to realize he was not there. I found myself going into his room to get him up for breakfast. I found myself going to his room on Sunday morning to lay out his nice clothes for church, only to realize he was not here. I found myself fixing him a plate of dessert at my mom's.

It was hard. There were many times I would start to breathe heavily, my heart would race, and I would begin to hyperventilate. I was on the verge of having a panic attack. Then I would take a deep breath and start claiming the scripture "Be anxious for nothing" in Philippians 4:6. I would calm down and go outside to walk around the house. I would look to heaven and ask Jesus to tell Mike "hello" and to tell him how much we missed him. Even the dog moped around the house for a few weeks. She would walk into Mike's room, glance around with a confused look, and then lie down.

The first weeks were awful. It was as though there was a huge hole in our lives that we would never fill up again, but we would eventually learn to live with the hole. The first church dinner without him was strange and sad. It will be hard at the first football games without him and the holidays will seem empty without him. I hope we do okay on December 16, his birthday. Maybe I can take a cake to his grave and blow out the candles, and play Pin the Tale on the Elephant. We have incredible memories that we will never forget.

As time passed, the days became more and more difficult. Not only had we lost Mike, but the house we had lived in for almost seventeen years was Mike's. Now that he was gone, the house was to be sold. Brad and I did not make enough money as a teacher and a janitor to afford to purchase a home like this one. It was scary. We had four children who needed a home. We knew God would take care of us, but it was hard not to worry.

Mike had said several times over the years, "I will fight for my family." He would say it during crazy times or trying times, and I always assumed he meant he would beat up anyone with his karate chops who tried to hurt us. One night, the pressure of losing him and possibly losing the house became too much. I walked outside and I could hear him in my mind saying, "I'll fight for my family." I pictured him in his room, on his knees, next to his bed with his hands folded and his eyes turned toward heaven saying to God, "I'll fight for my family." I suddenly knew what he meant. He knew that someday he would have to leave us, and that he had been praying that God would take care of us when he was gone. He had spent years "fighting for his family" on his knees. Now, he was gone. I realized that I would have to take over fighting for this family.

I started praying. I marched around the house and told Satan that he did not own this family and that God would take care of us. I have marched around the house seven times, and prayed every evening, since Mike died. I have no idea what God's plans are for us, but I know he cares for us and we will be okay.

Many people have come to us and said, "Your family gave Mike a wonderful life. It was a great thing you did. Mike was blessed to have you." We would swallow back the tears and reply, "Mike gave *us* a wonderful life. We are the ones who were blessed."

Kaylee came to me a few weeks after Mike had passed away and told me she had written a song about Mike. I sat on my bed and listened to my daughter sing from her heart the words of an incredible tribute to Mike. Notice the song never mentions Down's syndrome, yet it portrays Mike beautifully. The song went like this:

Dear Brother oh how we love you
You had the biggest heart I ever saw
You put everyone else above you.
And I know it hurt sometimes to be the way you were.
But, I am thankful for your mother's choice.
You must have meant the world to her.
I thank my God for sending you to us
You have no idea how much your joyful heart meant to all of us.

Chorus:
Mike you're the one who would smile no matter what
The one who brightened up my day.
The one who never knew a stranger?
Oh how you loved to pray

Mike you're the reason why we always laughed with joy
The reason for the smile on my face
You give me reason to thank my Lord every day for giving me life
Mike you're a hero
Dear Brother oh how we love you
You had a smile that melted hearts
I strive to be more like you

And I know you loved us so
It showed on your face.
You were our precious miracle
Thanks to God's amazing grace

Chorus
I would love to see you now
Dancing with joy
We miss you. We miss you
But we will see you soon

Life is very different without Mike. Our lives had changed forever on Halloween 1991. I would not change a single thing about keeping Mike. I can't wait to see him again; our little spook, our buddy, our son, our Mikey Spikey, our prayer warrior, our comedian, our biggest fan, and our friend.

Mike Williams Douthit

You are forever in our hearts.

See ya soon, good ol' buddy.

Epilogue

National statistics show that 95 percent of Down's syndrome babies are now being aborted in the United States. I assume society is trying to wipe out this race of human beings. It saddens me as I think of the incredible memories I have of Mike, and I ponder how richly people's lives could have been blessed if they would have allowed God to bless them with a Down's syndrome child. I am forever thankful to Mike's biological mother that she chose life.

On Sunday evening, October 25, 2009, (Grandma Dareing's 80th birthday), during the editing process of this book, we came home to find that our precious little dog, that absolutely adored Mike, had been ran over and killed. We buried her in our backyard under our "Mike Tree" that we planted after he passed away. It has been very difficult for us as it feels like another part of Mike is gone.

Famous Quotes
by Mike Williams Douthit

"Hamburger, French fries, Coke, please"

"You a good cook"

"I get married to Becky tomorrow"

"Watch it, BUSTER"

"Oh Lord, help her settle down"

"Bob did it!"

"He's Satan" (referring to Rick and Chris)

"I'm Deputy Sheriff"

"You so beautiful"

"MMMM … That's good"

"Mrs. Eads needs to whip her son"

"Hal-lay-loo-yuh!"

"Ain't that awful"

"Hey Toots"

"Oh, that makes me nervous"

"Oh, BULL!"

"She needs Jesus"

"I like that"

"You better believe it!"

"I'm hungry"

"I love you, Daddy darling"

115

"She went off like a Roman candle"

"My vacation on, already on"

"We go see the nice old people?"

"Sweeping, mopping, dusting"

"I'm pregnant, I'm gonna have a baby"

"I fight for my family"

"I sick my daddy on you!"

"You look like Barbara Bush"

"Honor your fadder and mudder"

"Thank you, Lord, this name to thee"

"There's two retards in this family"

"She retarded like me"

"We'll see time comes"

"Oh, come on!"

"You fight for me?"

"I'm a Republican!"

"You so sweet"

"I'm a Baptacostal!"

"I pray for you"

"Zeeeeeeekkke!!!"

"I know that"

"You crazy"

"You dodo head"

"My faucet's leaking"

"Howdy, partner"

"Thank the Lord"

"You so special"